Between the Covers

Between the Covers

Sexual freedom
through the bond of **Christian marriage**

Dr Christo Scheepers
& Dr Dainty Shaw

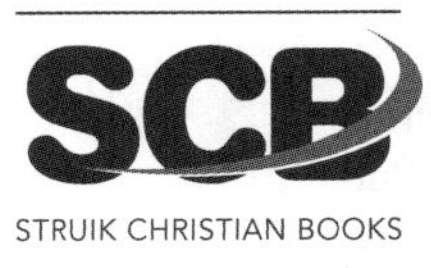

STRUIK CHRISTIAN BOOKS

BETWEEN THE COVERS

Published in 2012 by Struik Christian Books
An imprint of Struik Christian Media
A division of New Holland Publishing (South Africa) (Pty) Ltd
(New Holland Publishing is a member of Avusa Ltd.)
Wembley Square, First Floor
Solan Street, Gardens
Cape Town, 8001

Reg. No. 1971/009721/07

Unless otherwise indicated, Scripture quotations are from *The Amplified Bible* (AMP) © 1987, Zondervan Publishing House; *The Holy Bible*, New International Version (NIV) © 1984, International Bible Society; *The Holy Bible*, New King James Version (NKJV) © 1982, Thomas Nelson, Inc.

Disclaimer
This book is designed to provide condensed information. It is not intended to reprint all the information that is otherwise available, but instead to complement, amplify and supplement other texts. You are urged to read all the available material, learn as much as possible and tailor the information to your individual needs. Every effort has been made to make this book as complete and as accurate as possible. However, there may be mistakes, both typographical and in content. Therefore, this text should be used only as a general guide and not as the ultimate source of information. The purpose of this book is to educate. The authors and publisher shall have neither liability nor responsibility to any person or entity with respect to any loss or damage caused, or alleged to have been caused, directly or indirectly, by the information contained in this book.

Project management by Elzanne Loest
Edited by Glynne Newlands
Cover design and DTP by Sonja Louw
Illustrations by Astrid Castle
Cover image from Shutterstock
Printed and bound by Paarl Media,
Jan van Riebeeck Drive, Paarl, South Africa

ISBN 978-1-4153-1304-6 (Print)
ISBN 978-1-4153-2056-3 (ePub)
ISBN 978-1-4153-2054-9 (PDF)

www.struikchristianmedia.co.za

Acknowledgements

Thank you to my dear husband, Joris, and my beautiful daughters, Vicky and Denise, for your support.

I would like to thank my dear friend Christo for inviting me to write this book with him. He is a professional mentor, being patient, persistent, knowledgeable and very kind, even with the challenge of writing together over a great distance, different working hours and communication hurdles. Thank you and bless you, Christo.

Thank you to everyone who has ever believed in my capabilities and who enjoys it when I reach my goals. I really enjoyed writing this book knowing that marriages will be blessed. Thank you and bless you.

All glory to the Kingdom.

Dainty

Thank you to my Lord and Saviour, Jesus Christ, for believing in me when no-one else had any faith left in me. You were always ready to lift me up again after I fell and You were always willing to give me a second chance. Praise You, God of the second chance.

Christo

Thank you to Mr. David Shaw for proofreading this manuscript and for your valuable feedback.

Dainty & Christo

Contents

Foreword

WARNING – very sexy book! Proceed with caution!

Between the Covers is a no-nonsense, practical book, encouraging sexual experimentation within the safety of marriage in a godly way. Both authors are frank about their own experiences, displaying a vulnerability that I hope will transfer to you, the reader, as you explore sexual issues with your spouse.

As a therapist for more than 25 years, I see many clients struggling with sexual issues. Some have embraced various addictive or perverted sexual practices in a desperate attempt to come to terms with their sexuality. Others, terrified of being inadequate and/or ignorant in the sexual arena, have withdrawn or chosen to tolerate sex. Yet God wants us to enjoy and celebrate sex. Wouldn't it be wonderful if in a pre-marriage counselling setting the counsellor or pastor handed over this book and said, 'Read *Between the Covers* and then we can talk!'?

This book explains the act of sex, sexuality, dysfunctions, the effects of personality and so much more, in a way that is easy to understand. But don't negate the simplicity of this book!

Many clients who are about to be married have come to me in tears and frightened because they have no idea how to pleasure their soon-to-be spouse in the bedroom. Instead of looking forward to their honeymoon as an exciting, wonderful, climactic (pardon the pun) time, they dread it and wrap it up in fear, anxiety, poor technique and everything that God did not intend sex to be.

I often hear questions like these below, and maybe you have wondered about the answers:

- Can we only use the missionary position or will it be acceptable to try something else? (Will God approve? Is it perverted to try something else?)
- How do I give my husband oral sex?
- Do I have to?!
- Is it hygienic to even put your mouth 'there'? (trying to find reasons to avoid having oral sex)
- We're two consenting adults; why can't we whip each other and get into some sadism and masochism? Surely all we need is to be consenting? It's not like one is forcing themselves on the other!
- What do I actually do in bed?
- What about sex toys? Does God 'allow' that?
- What turns my wife/husband on? I have no idea.

Between the Covers answers these questions — and more.

What I like about *Between the Covers* is that it doesn't seek to crack a peanut with an atom bomb. The instructions are simple, yet eloquent. The subject matter is complex, yet easy to understand.

In the church we find well-intentioned parents telling their children 'Don't have sex. It's wrong!' Now we know that this is a valid statement from parents wanting to protect their children from soul ties, but the confusion arises when these same children grow up and are at the threshold of marriage. These parents now tell their young adults, 'Have sex. Sex is good. It is the glue in your marriage.' No wonder there is so much confusion and angst around sex in the church today!

Bishop Frank Retief likes to say, 'You can be sincere; but you can be sincerely wrong'. And this is certainly a case for being sincerely wrong.

For many years I worked in correctional centres and observed some dysfunctional attitudes pertaining to sex – besides the overt ones around paedophilia, rape, incest and the like. One of these was in the area of homosexuality. Inmates believed that having sex with a man was a necessary thing when incarcerated, but it did not mean that the inmates were homosexual! In fact, one of the numbers gangs go so far as to have a 'silver line', which is a group of men set aside exclusively to service the rest of the gang members sexually. These men are called '*wyfies.*' In this specific gang, being a *wyfie* is their 'calling' and they just accept that it is what it is. But there are consequences to this… soul ties, objectifying the bride of Christ, being an abomination in the eyes of God and the onslaught of HIV/AIDS.

In correctional centres the HIV rate is approximately seven percent higher than 'outside'. A lot of the gangs use rape, sodomy and the like as gang initiation rites.

So, today, I believe that you have picked up this book for a very specific reason and for a very exact purpose. You are holding a tool in your hand that will change your sex life and your thought life forever. The practical information and questionnaires will set you on a new path. May you burn with the passionate fire that God has placed inside you and unleash the wild child within you!

Dr. Lesly Uys (D.Th. Counselling)
– Addictions & Marriage Counsellor

You must be thinking: Am I okay with my wife writing a sexual book of this nature with another man? The answer is yes. I am truly impressed. A book of this nature has long been needed in book stores nationwide; the book opens communication between a husband and wife, is based on Christian principles and it can release the wild child between them. The secret formula lies in the depth of the book, and we hope it will prevent divorce and broken marriages, of which there are such high percentages worldwide.

Joris Shaw, Tender Procurement Consultant

Between the Covers is an excellent book on teaching couples how to have satisfying sex and how to bring out the wild child in the lives of married couples. I like the godly factor in the book and the way it portrays how God intends sex to be enjoyed within the boundaries of marriage. God can use this excellent guide to save marriages. It will help couples to fan the flame in their marriages and to re-encounter God in their marriages and sex lives. It is a must-have for your bookshelf.

Teresa K. Scheepers, B.Th.

This book is well worth reading and is sure to keep you riveted, as a high-class mystery or suspense work does. As a medical doctor, I find the book a timely and refreshing new approach to a deep-seated and unnervingly huge problem in marriages in our country. I recommend it as a must-have wedding present to be given as early as possible to help such a glorious relationship develop into what God meant it to be.

Dr. Dirk J. Brink, MB.ChB. [Pretoria], General Practitioner

Author preface

Dr. R. Dainty Shaw

Shalom to you. Thank you for choosing this book; it will bless you as you apply it to your life. My husband and I have a good and loving marriage with privileges and challenges founded in the Christian faith.

Joris and I have been together for 22 years and married each other three times during this time! In the first two marriages we were saved but not living changed lives. There were many trials and tribulations; we had to call on God and listen to the Holy Spirit before the third marriage finally worked successfully.

My studies in counselling greatly contributed to growth and maturity towards the Kingdom way of living. It is my hope that sharing the knowledge and insight God put in my life enriches your sexual life.

It would give me great joy to discover that you have been blessed with the knowledge and insight in this book, to the glory of the Kingdom of God.

Kingdom love,

Dr. Dainty

Dr. Christo A. Scheepers

Hi, my name is Christo. I am the analytical one, always speaking directly, and I want to thank you for taking the time to read this book which promises to change your marital sex life forever. How, you may ask? You will have to come with us on this journey through Christian sexuality as we take you on a wild ride towards God's intended plan for sex in marriage.

I grew up loving the Lord and gave my heart to Him at the age of 11 in a Sunday school class, but only gave my whole life to Him in January 1999 while studying Christian Counselling. I had a radical born-again experience and was filled with the Holy Spirit. I experienced his anointing and call on my life to help people grow from trauma to triumph, and thus ended up as an internationally ordained minister of the Gospel with a Doctorate in Interdisciplinary Studies and a qualified Doctor of Natural Medicine; since then I have offered trauma debriefing and trauma counselling to hundreds of people. Especially in the area of sexual and marital trauma.

The need for a book like this has been seen in the consulting room and therefore we attempt to provide you with some information to use for your benefit and marital bliss.

So if you dare, take this awesome journey towards sexual fulfilment in marriage and let us be your facilitators in guiding you towards fulfilled sexuality in marriage.

Jesus love,

Christo

Introduction

Between the Covers was birthed from the obvious lack of available resources and the lack of sexual fulfilment in marriages, confirmed by the high divorce rate and the numerous affairs married people are having.

When people experience marital problems, they are often carried over into the bedroom, leading to sexually frustrated and unfulfilled couples. This is evident in modern-day society and characterised by either extramarital affairs or very unhappy people longing for more action in the bedroom.

Even if you or your spouse have never been involved in an extramarital affair, the question still remains whether you are fully satisfied sexually. Are you truly fulfilled with your sex life or are you longing for more, but do not know how to share this yearning with your spouse? Do you want to try something new in the bedroom, but fear rejection? Are you having difficulty adjusting to your spouse's sexual cycle and need for sex?

If you answer yes to any of these questions, then you should continue reading and even take the next step: inviting your spouse to share in reading *Between the Covers.*

The purpose of *Between the Covers* is to make you aware of the inner passion within you. We believe that every man and woman has sexual passion inside them, but it may have been suppressed due to circumstances, fear, rejection, past sexual experiences, negative connotations to sexual pleasure or sexual abuse. Allow us to facilitate the process of discovering the passion inside you and unleashing this inner sexual need within the confines of marriage so that you may also experience sex as God intended it to be from the very beginning.

In *Between the Covers* you will discover what true sexuality was meant to be, based on the godly plan revealed in the Word of God. You will discover how to deal with dormant sexual desires while involving your spouse in this exciting journey towards sexual fulfilment. Most important of all, you will learn how to become compatible with your spouse's sexual needs and desires while giving each other the non-judgemental platform in the bedroom to unleash each other's passion, thus giving your spouse the opportunity to be a truly whole person.

Why would two people who are not married to each other write a book of this nature together, you may ask? Well, most books on sexuality are written either by married couples or professionals (usually of the same gender and of the same opinions). This causes a tendency to portray a specific couple's opinion of sexual matters or a certain professional opinion. This may result in a very one-sided or limited point of view, sometimes seen as very judgemental towards people who differ in opinion.

With two friends of different genders writing *Between the Covers* together, you are assured of a well-balanced point of view on sexual matters. We offer you the opinions, backgrounds and experiences of different people and couples. As authors we both agree on the crucial matter of believing in Jesus Christ as our Lord and Saviour no matter what our past experiences entail. This foundation is strengthened by our professional backgrounds in counselling.

As you can imagine, when friends of different genders write a book of this nature together, very personal information is shared and discussed and as born-again Christians, we embarked on this project with two very definite policies; firstly to have our spouses' blessing on the project and being open to discuss anything coming up with our respective spouses, and secondly to protect and keep confidential the other's sensitive information. True to our confidential nature in the counselling profession, this was a natural outflow of common courtesy.

The interesting part was learning from another married couple very intimate details about sexuality while comparing it to your own relationship. The challenging part was to openly and honestly share very intimate sexual details about your own life and marriage. The enlightening part was becoming conscious of the truth of the Word of God when applied to sexuality, and the positive influence it has on your own sexual life, and releasing your inner passion when looking at a Scripture like John 8:32, which states that you will know the Truth and the Truth will set you free.

The Truth mentioned in this Scripture refers to Jesus and since He is the Truth, getting to know Him is what sets a person free. When your relationship with Jesus develops and you draw closer to Him on a daily basis, you soon realise that the past cannot be changed and the future is yet to come, but how you live in the present is what will determine your future. When you live in the present in a godly way, you become aware of how important it is to enjoy every single moment of your life. You soon realise there is no reason to hide your sexual needs and desires from your spouse; you can be honest enough to discuss them with your partner, regardless of how uncomfortable it makes you feel.

Do not fool yourself; it might be very uncomfortable at first because some of us have grown up where sex is not something we talk about or parents teach their children that sex is dirty in an attempt to keep them from exploring at a too young age. That being said, children today find it much easier to talk about sex and do not see any problem with multiple sexual partners due to what the media is suggesting. This is, however, not the case for the older generation who still see sex as taboo. But the reality is that this approach is totally ineffective – you look at the current pregnancy rate of teenagers and the rate at which abortions are performed on a daily basis. So if this approach is totally ineffective in keeping teenagers from having premarital sex, what is it doing? The obvious answer is that it is causing people to suppress their sexual desires instead of effectively dealing with them in a godly way. It is causing teenagers to view sex as something to hide from their parents and other people, resulting in these incorrect beliefs being carried over into their marriages which can lead to innumerable sexual problems inside the confines of marriage.

What is the answer then? We believe that when parents honestly and openly teach godly principles and moral values to their children from an appropriate age, they will be able to make the correct decisions about premarital sex instead of just getting involved in it without their parents' knowledge. When parents take up their godly responsibility to share the Truth with their children and live as godly role-models, their children will grow up with a deep-seated knowing of who they are in Jesus Christ and experience a godly dignity, thus setting them up to make decisions based on the Word of God instead of peer pressure. When they know who they are, they will not have to get approval from their peers to feel good about themselves and this will lead to moral and godly decisions.

As a result, these teenagers will grow up and get married to the right spouses instead of settling for ungodly partners. They will then be able to truly experience sexual fulfilment in their marriages and live out their sexuality within the safety and confines of marriage, thus reducing the risk of HIV, sexually transmitted diseases (STDs) and emotional pain and hurt. As whole people, they will be able to unleash their inner passions in marriage.

Unleashing your inner passion has been mentioned a few times now, but what exactly is meant by this? It can be said that every person has a 'naughty' side; a so-called inner sexual passion. This is a side often suppressed due to past experiences, wrong beliefs taught to us since childhood and fear of rejection if our spouses find out.

Is this inner passion thus a side of perversion and sin? No, definitely not! It is a side every person and married couple should embrace, to take their sexuality from mediocre to extraordinary. It is the playful side that often becomes dormant as we grow up and take on more and more responsibility; the effortless side forced into hibernation in order for the responsible adult to emerge. Unleashing your inner passion is getting in touch with this playful side again, but especially in the area of your sexuality. When your inner passion is unleashed, you will be able to combine marital sex with playfulness and be able to experience your sexuality as a wonderful part of yourself and your marriage without seeing sex as a marital duty to perform. It will change your sex life from an obligation to a game, a delightful and intimate pastime making God smile on your marriage.

Sex was never intended to be a duty or only something to be done to procreate. If it was, God would never have made it such a pleasurable experience. God gave sex to be used within the boundaries of marriage for husbands and wives to enjoy each other and share their love with each other in a very intimate and pleasurable way. Yes, it was also intended for married couples to procreate and produce children, the ultimate result of their love for each other, but it was never for reproduction only.

'God Himself invented sex for our delight. It was his gift to us – *intended for pleasure.*'[1] 'It was God who invented sex. The devil is incapable of creative powers. His purpose is to destroy, corrupt and defile that which is good.'[2] 'We would indeed displease God if we associated every need for sexual fulfilment with sin.'[3]

Looking at these statements, it is evident that God gave sex to married couples to enjoy each other and not only for reproduction. It is furthermore confirmed by the Word of God in Genesis 2:25 where it says, 'And the man and his wife were both naked and were not embarrassed *or* ashamed in each other's presence'. It should be clearly noted this Scripture mentions a husband and wife being naked and comfortable in each other's company; this was all before sin even entered the world. God gave sex for husbands and wives to get pleasure from each other and the more comfortable, honest and open you are with your spouse, the more enjoyable and satisfying sex will be.

Coming from this premise of sex being a godly gift to married couples, *Between the Covers* was written from a Christian perspective and from an experiential environment instead of being a medical textbook on the subject of sex.

We invite you to accompany us on this sexual journey of unleashing your inner passion and discovering again the pleasures of sex within your marriage. As far as possible, we will avoid professional jargon and we will openly and honestly talk to you about sexual fulfilment. So, make the decision now to involve your spouse as you both buckle up for this straight-to-the-point ride of unleashing the inner passion hidden inside each of you.

CHAPTER 1

Laying the foundation

Unleashing your inner sexual passion is a journey every married couple should embark on to release playfulness in the bedroom. Discover the joy of sexual teasing and experimentation while enjoying each other without being bound by preconceived ideas and wrong beliefs about marital sexuality.

Sex should not be viewed as a carnal sin, but as part of the innermost being of every human. Some cultures, even today, view sexuality as sacred and connected to spirituality. We believe humans have been created with intertwining dimensions of which the sexual dimension plays an equal part. Sexuality being part of the spiritual dimension is therefore not a strange concept at all.

Consequently, what the Bible has to say about sexuality should play a major part in laying the foundation of unleashing your inner passion. Chapter 2 has been set aside for viewing the biblical foundation of this process.

Laying the foundation for unleashing your inner passion is therefore more practical in nature, while the following chapter will focus more on the biblical aspects of the subject.

The foundation consists of the basic building blocks necessary to create the correct ambience for releasing your inhibitions in the bedroom. Making this a reality should never be seen as a task to accomplish, but rather as a game to play and enjoy.

Sex should be fun!

In many circles sex is seen as something sinister and something never to speak about, but sex was never intended to be categorised as such. Sex is something most people think about and are curious about, but due to social taboos and preconceived ideas, sex is rarely openly talked about.

The need is therefore evident to lay a solid foundation for married couples to enter into a process of unleashing an inner passion possibly suppressed by society, background and cultural expectations.

Having your sexual passion unleashed while encouraging your spouse to do the same is not seen as optional, but as a necessity in every marriage and therefore all suppressing causes should be overcome to ensure you experience a sex life for which you have been intended and designed.

It is so easy to fall into a rut of settling for substandard sex, especially if you are not even aware that you have the right to unleash your inner sexual passion and live out your inner desires within your marriage. In the counselling room we often see how the lack of satisfactory sex is the reason for break-ups; these couples are not usually aware of having the right to enjoy sex and live out their deepest sexual desires within the marriage.

A few basic building blocks are essential for the unleashing of your inner sexual passion so that when it is set free, it is unleashed appropriately within an accommodating environment.

1.1 Playfulness

The first building block to lay in unleashing your inner passion is playfulness. Try not to take life so seriously that it begins to affect your sexual life, forcing your inner passion into hibernation or a boring sex life.

Spouses should enjoy each other. They should become comfortable with their own sexuality, extending it to their spouses by teasing each other, playing with each other and just enjoying the others' company.

Viewing sex as a two-player game to be enjoyed is the first step in releasing playfulness in the bedroom that will inevitably lead to enjoyment and seeing sex as fun. This is the ultimate goal spouses should aim towards; enjoying sex!

Sex was never intended to become a secret never to be discussed; it was designed to be a crucial release of tension and the best fun spouses should have with each other.

When spouses realise the importance of sex in marriage, they will begin to pay more attention to it. They will move away from hiding away their sexuality to the revealing of their inner passion to their spouses. Society should no longer restrain you from being the whole person you are supposed to be; no longer should sex be seen as taboo, but within the safety of your marriage you should fully release your sexuality and make your spouse the happiest married person imaginable!

See sex as fun and when you begin to enjoy sex, your spouse will follow your lead and the two of you can become so sexually fulfilled within your marriage that it will naturally lead to more playfulness between you for days, months and years to follow.

Parents often portray, sex as something to hide or to be ashamed of in an attempt to prolong the innocence of teenagers. A noble effort, but the long-term results are usually the suppression of sexuality and inner sexual passion. This is not a real issue until it is carried into marriage. When you are married and your spouse wants to explore you sexually but you are full of inhibitions, it is usually the first sign of reality versus passion. When your spouse wants you to initiate the sexual exploration but you are too reserved to even attempt the expedition, you should realise something is preventing you from releasing your inner sexual passion in the bedroom and that intervention is needed.

Playfulness with your spouse, combined with teasing and fun, should be the very basic requirements to meet when intervention is needed.

When a couple has established sex as fun and playful recreational activity, they will not only be able to enjoy their time together and their sexuality much more, they will also be able to put down other building blocks in laying the foundation of unleashing their inner passion.

1.2 Mental viewpoint

Your mental viewpoint is all about your worldview and how you perceive certain things in life. How do you view marriage? How do you see sex? These are the types of questions that can be answered by the way you think.

To unleash your inner sexual passion, you need to first consider your viewpoint on marriage and sexuality. Various viewpoints exist, ranging from viewing the husband as king, priest and prophet in the marriage to viewing the wife as a doormat. These viewpoints are so varied and numerous that we do not intend to change your view, but rather to challenge it and offer you a biblical alternative you might want to consider. Why, you may ask? Well, we want to lay the best possible foundation in your life and marriage to facilitate the unleashing of your inner passion.

You may believe that your husband should be the leader, the minister and the one giving direction. This is a valid biblical position, but from a very conservative theological position. This viewpoint is especially followed in certain cultures where women are often seen as doormats who should submit to their husbands in everything based on Scriptural reference.[4] Sometimes this position is abused to the point where the husband expects the wife to agree with everything he wants. When this happens, it is very unhealthy because it does not take into consideration the preceding Scripture saying husbands and wives should be subject to one another[5] and not only the wife to the husband.

This is exactly the viewpoint we want to introduce you to; where the husband and wife love each other and submit to each other. This viewpoint does not portray the wife as less valuable and important than the husband, but rather that they are of equal importance. To put this in very practical terms, let us consider the household chores agreed upon by the husband and wife. They might have agreed the wife will take care of the dirty dishes while the husband will take care of the lawn; very traditional in many cultures, but workable. So what happens when the wife is ill? Based on the misperceptions accompanying the position of the husband being the king, priest and prophet, the husband will still expect the wife to clean the dishes since he will see himself as too superior to involve him in such a 'female' task. The viewpoint we are suggesting is an equal partnership where the husband will assist the wife in cleaning the dishes when she is ill, but also when she is not in an attempt to spend more time with each other.

The equal partnership approach is one of love, where the husband and wife are seen as equals in the marriage, where each has a valid opinion to be taken into consideration and, when decisions are to be taken, it is not left to the husband, but after discussion they should both agree on the way forward. When this viewpoint is followed, the husband and wife are both involved in decision making and the way forward is preceded by full agreement of both spouses.

Spouses should love one another regardless of shortcomings and possible traditional gender roles and functions at work in their marriage. Spouses should help each other complete household chores even when they are not necessarily part of traditional gender roles. Wives may assist their husbands in the garden and washing the car while husbands help wives to do the laundry or wash the dishes. In this way, they will spend additional time together and, in the process, reduce the load on each other, increasing the desire for sex. One thing to remember: when your spouse helps you with a task, accept it as a gift without finding fault and making negative remarks about the way the task is being done. Just because your spouse is not doing something in exactly the way you do, is no reason for you to reject the help and ultimately your spouse in the process.

Your mental viewpoint will often direct the unleashing of your inner passion, especially when it comes to the way you view your spouse and how your spouse views you. When you see your spouse as a valuable gift from God, you will be able to behave and act towards him or her in a more appropriate manner.

Never treat your spouse as a doormat, as someone to be mistreated or to be overloaded with household chores while you are off doing whatever you want to do. Never make your spouse feel insecure or abused. Do not take your spouse for granted, but always put in every effort to make him or her feel valuable.

Self-image and the way you see yourself is the responsibility of every individual, but when you are married, your spouse's opinion and behaviour towards you has a direct influence on the way you see yourself. You, therefore, have an important part to play in how you see yourself, your spouse and your marriage, and if you want to see the inner sexual passion unleashed in your spouse, begin to edify instead of humiliate. You might be surprised how easily the inner passion in your spouse is unleashed when you take it upon yourself to make your spouse feel good about him or herself at all times.

Your viewpoint should be founded in love and respect.

1.3 Atmosphere

What is the atmosphere like in your house? Is it an atmosphere of peace, calmness and serenity or rather an atmosphere of strife, bickering and unhappiness?

Every house and every marriage has an atmosphere and that atmosphere is directly related to the state of the marriage. The atmosphere of your marriage will also determine the unleashing of your inner sexual passion or the suppression thereof.

Try to create an atmosphere of love and respect for your spouse in which both of you can freely unleash your inner passion. Generally women tend to long more for love while men tend to need respect, but ultimately both men and women need love and respect.

1.4 The bedroom

1.4.1 The bed

You are going to enjoy this chapter and in a minute you will see why. When I was a child I used to walk to my parent's bedroom in the mornings and nestle there until it was time to get up. I remember how comfy the bed was and how snugly the linen wrapped itself around me.

When I think back on it, I also remember my mom mention that they bought the bed when they were newly-weds. Later my mom and dad divorced and the bed stayed with my dad and his second wife. I realised the same bed must have been in use for about 37 years. Our family believed in the principle that if it is working, it does not need fixing or replacing, only regular cleaning and polishing. Astonishing! However, I now think differently. I change my bed at least every five years because I spend a third of my life in bed and feel I deserve it!

I have no idea how old your bed is and if it is anything older than five years, with your spouse's agreement I give you permission to get rid of it and get a new one! Are you enjoying this chapter already? Thought so!

Just before you run out the door, remember to take this book with you as we need to discuss a few other options. Beds are sold like hamburgers; there are plenty of choices to suit every individual's personal taste, so you need to figure out what it is you and your spouse prefer. Does he like a long base for his long legs, does she like a firm base for better back support, how big or small should your bed be? Double beds are your most common choice, like a basic cheeseburger with no garnish and no sauces. First and foremost, you and your spouse must be able to get a good night's sleep of an average of eight hours per night. You can ask a sales assistant to explain to you the variations in beds, as this will help you to decide. Secondly, but no less important, is whether the bed will serve the purpose of making love on it.

Do you remember sleeping on grandma's bed? It squeaked as if it wanted to wake up the whole neighbourhood! When you wanted to turn you had to wrap the blankets around your arms and legs in one quick turn and then turn and lie still until the next morning. When you wanted to go to the toilet, you'd have to roll off the bed instead of sitting up to shuffle off the bed! So guys, don't buy a bed that will squeak in the next five years, especially when you are planning to have great sex on it. The only noise around should be you and your spouse's echoes of desire.

So now you have a great bed for a good night's rest and great sex! Let's make the bed. What linen do you like? The choices are wide but a first choice should be sleeping between white cotton sheets. Both white and cotton are good to look at and healthy against your skin when you sweat, sleep or rub against, plus it is easy to clean. You might want to consider the option of silky sheets when your spouse and finances agree. It is something different from the usual and you have plenty of colours from which to choose. Remember to change sheets and pillow cases regularly.

Some individuals prefer sleeping under a blanket and on a sheet or the other way around. It does not matter how you sleep in your bed; it is important to get a good night's rest. When your linen makes you sweat or shiver every night, you might feel tired every morning. Maybe the solution is as simple as changing your bedding.

Couples have different ways of making their bedrooms comfortable. Some people do not mind clothes and shoes lying around, and others do not mind the family pet sleeping on the bed. Some couples barely move while they sleep. How ever you prefer your bedroom to be, it is important that both spouses should be happy with how your bedroom looks. Remember God is first in your life and then your spouse, not the bed, the dog, the washing, perfection or the TV. It is also important for you to look after your rest and then your marriage. So if the dog takes preference in there, it's time the dog gets its own space somewhere else.

A couple who were married for several years once complained because the one took on stray pets and let them all sleep on the bed to the extent their spouse had no rest, a lot of discomfort and sometimes had to move over so one of the pets could sleep next to their spouse. This might be your situation. If so, you need to look at the situation and assess whether it is good for you and your spouse's health and marriage.

Spouses should *not* share their bed with anything but each other. Not a pillow in between, a pet, a child or teddy bear.

For both spouses, touch during the night is of great importance towards good health, except where the couple are unintentionally keeping each other awake through muscle twitching on hands or feet, regular nightmares or the like. The necessity of sleeping apart does not indicate a divorce on the horizon and should spouses decide to do this, they have to make more effort to build their bond together as one. Remember to make it clear to your children. Their security depends on your marriage and stability. If they understand you need separate beds for a good night's rest and that you will sleep together when the occasion arises, they'll realise that this practice need not apply to their marriage some day.

Making love should be easier now that you are organised with a bed, nice linen and nothing in the bed except for your spouse!

Most hotels and lodges focus on curtains with a thick back curtain to keep the sunlight out and many different small lights in the bedroom to provide lighting. It is a great idea to have the option of having sunlight in your room in the mornings or not.

Mid-summer and mid-winter months can be very uncomfortable to make love, so you might want to consider an excellent air-conditioning unit or maybe something cheaper like an electric blanket with two controls, a heater with a remote or a fan. It'll be more relaxing keeping your room at room temperature while making love.

The colour of your room is important as some colours create energy and others relax. We recommend relaxing colours which includes all earthy and very soft colours. You can create the necessary energy through lingerie. Discuss the matter with your spouse and plan ahead for something really nice to wear in red, green, even gold and silver or blue. Keep in mind your spouse may appreciate a surprise.

1.4.2 Accessories in the bedroom

This book aims to inform you on how to benefit as much as you can from your sexual relationship with your spouse. We share what we have learnt and experienced through life but it is and stays your choice whether you want to make use of the information.

I suggest getting rid of all the clutter and leave only the basics, such as the furniture or the mosquito net. So you might want to get a box to pack everything into! Any bedroom can look extremely beautiful with the right curtains, bedding and a few things like a couch and a tray for coffee and tea.

Love me afterwards. Your bedroom is the place where your mind, emotions and spirit should be able to come to rest and at will, have great sexual pleasure and serve God. You can pack away the mirror too. The only time a brain relaxes is when the eyes do not have to look and assess anything. The unconscious mind does not know the difference between reality and fantasy; both are real to the unconscious mind. In your bedroom, you can read your Bible, you can have great sex, you can get on your knees and pray, you can scratch your spouse's back or you can make him or her a cup of tea.

Since we have a tendency to nest into our bedroom, open the windows and let the sunlight in on a regular basis.

We suggest that you and your spouse go to bed at the same time and wake up at the same time, but we are all different, so don't push yourself to do this; it is merely suggestion to be able to build on your sexual relationship.

Your bedroom should be a peaceful pleasure for you and your spouse to enjoy your rest, enjoy each other and spend time with God.

1.5 Unleashing communication

Communication between spouses is one of the most important building blocks when laying the foundation for the release of your inner sexual passion. In fact, it is so important a whole chapter has been set aside to deal with communication in more depth, but here we are specifically going to look at how to unleash communication with your spouse.

The importance of communication can never be underestimated; it is the way two people share their thoughts and dreams with each other. It is the way spouses deal with their differences and it is the manner in which spouses share their love and passion with each other.

The ability to communicate with your spouse is the basic requirement for a healthy marriage, a healthy relationship and the unleashing of your inner passion. If not for communication, how will your spouse know what you want and how will you know what your spouse likes or dislikes? Without effective communication between you there is no way for either of you to know exactly what the other one wants, needs and longs for.

Effective communication is the ability to share with your spouse exactly what is happening inside you. It is the ability to inform your spouse what you require and long for sexually without being shy. It is the method of clearly and without reservation sharing with your spouse your inner desires, knowing that you will not be made fun of or humiliated, but rather accommodated within your marriage and so experience true sexual fulfilment while your inner passions are fully unleashed.

1.5.1 Overcoming shyness

Effective communication is only possible if you do not allow shyness to keep you from sharing your inner yearnings with your spouse. Shyness is an obstacle to be dealt with if it is going to lead your inner passion into hibernation.

Shyness is not only an obstacle when it comes to communication, but also when one spouse feels shy about his or her body, or one is shy about leaving the light on, or one wants to experiment with something but does not know how to share the desire with their spouse.

Dealing with shyness is of the utmost importance. Trying to determine where it originated is one of the first steps in overcoming it. Shyness may be the result of others making fun of you or it may have forced its way upon you when you tried something unconventional and it backfired. You may be naturally shy while your upbringing and experiences during your formative years might have added to it. You therefore have to determine where your shyness comes from. Tell your spouse about your shyness and that you are trying to deal with it, and ask for their assistance in the process. In this way your spouse will fully support you and you will not feel rejected or left out.

Once you have discovered the source of your shyness, clearly communicate it to your spouse and try to deal with it appropriately in order to overcome it. If you do not know how to deal with it effectively, it may be a good idea to approach a professional for assistance.

Shyness is sometimes linked to a bad self-image and you will have to deal with your self-image regardless of whether shyness is directly or indirectly linked to it, because it will also have an effect on the way you communicate with your spouse. Read the Bible and begin to build your self-image on the Word of God instead of on what others had to say about you or what you believe about yourself. Believe the Creator's opinion about you instead of allowing misconceptions to negatively influence the way you see yourself.

The Bible has plenty to say about your uniqueness and value in the eyes of God. Let us look at some Scriptures to see how valuable you are:

- You are the temple of the Holy Spirit[6]
- You are forgiven of all your sins you ever committed in the past if you just own up to it[7]
- You are a saint[8]
- You are the elect of God[9]
- You have been set free by this truth of God[10]
- You are more than a conqueror[11]
- You are free from condemnation[12]
- You are reconciled to God as His son or daughter.

These are just a few of the things the Bible has to say about who you are and how God sees you. You are valuable in the eyes of God.

What others say about you is therefore of secondary importance, because the primary and superior opinion has already been given by God.

When you begin to see yourself through the eyes of God and not through the opinions of religion, you will be set free like never before while your self-image will increase to a healthy level. Just to be clear: the difference between God's opinion and that of religion is based on what each stands for. God is the Creator and He is reaching out to you and all you have to do is to accept Him into your life and begin to build a relationship with Him. Religion, on the other hand, is man's attempt to reach out to God. We are of the opinion that God reaches out to marriages to set us free from all the religious rules and regulations placed on married couples by culture, society and people's ideas in order to bring freedom to marriages, to enjoy life and especially to enjoy your sexuality.

Realising all of this inevitably leads to spouses overcoming their shyness in order to increase intimacy and unleash passion.

1.5.2 How do you communicate your inner passions and desires?
Communication with your spouse should always be open and honest; having said that, always remember to communicate your inner passions and desires without causing offence or hurt.

When talking to your spouse about your deep desires and inner passions, try to do so in an atmosphere of love and respect while taking care not to offend, humiliate or make your spouse feel inadequate.

Be honest and speak openly with your spouse about what you would like to try and experiment with, but always from a personal perspective instead of attacking your spouse. In other words, use an approach where you say something like, 'I would like to try this because I have an inner need to fulfil this in order to feel alive'. This approach is a much more effective way of communicating instead of saying something like, 'We are going to do this, because if you do not allow me to, I am going to do it with somebody else.' This second approach is definitely done from a position lacking in respect and should never be used with your spouse.

1.5.3 How do you unleash your inner passion?
We have been talking about unleashing your inner passion, but how should this be done?

It is firstly discovering what exactly you want in the bedroom and then secondly effectively sharing this with your spouse from a perspective of love and respect. When you have told your spouse about your inner passion, listen to your spouse's inner passion and then come to an agreement as to how the two of you are going to make these desires a reality for each other. Once you have made a decision about how it will work for both of you and with which both of you are comfortable, you may continue with the most important step in unleashing your inner passion:

Practise, practise and practise! Enjoy every minute of this process.

1.6 Mental blocks

Mental blocks can be obstacles on the journey towards unleashing your inner passion. These are things holding you back and bind you in such a way that you are unable to let loose and make your inner desires a reality in your marriage.

There are many different mental blocks but we will only discuss the most obvious ones. You owe it to yourself and your spouse not to allow any mental blocks in your marriage which may prevent you from experiencing an unleashed sex life.

Overcoming mental blocks is a three-step process:

- Own up to the mental block and acknowledge its presence in your life.
- Determine how it entered your life, when it happened and what else happened during your life at that specific time period.
- Put a plan of action in place with your spouse's assistance in how you are going to overcome it.

Mental blocks are mostly overcome by facing them instead of ignoring them. When they are acknowledged and faced, they can be dealt with one by one in a way with which you are comfortable. If you are unable to deal with them effectively, you may want to consider seeking professional help.

1.6.1 Unforgiveness

Unforgiveness is possibly the biggest mental block of all because it affects you exactly where it hurts most. Unforgiveness usually comes from an injustice committed against you, causing deep hurt and pain. Every person experiencing unforgiveness has a valid reason to feel the way they do, but holding on to it only causes them to miss out on life.

When you feel unforgiveness towards someone who might have mistreated you in some way, they are possibly not even aware of your feelings so the only ones you are really negatively affecting by clinging on to it are yourself and your spouse.

This mental block is therefore overcome by recognising it and realising the negative effect it has on you. Then you should make the conscious decision to forgive the person. You may not feel like you want to, but you have to make the decision and decide to forgive. Once done, go ahead and forgive. It is a simple process during which you basically say aloud that you are forgiving the specific person for what he or she did to you and you fully release them to God.

Forgiving is not an easy process and the perpetrator might not even deserve forgiveness, but you should realise the importance of forgiving, because you are doing it for yourself and your marriage. In some cases you may want to physically go to the person and forgive, but that is not always necessary.

The other side of unforgiveness is also to be dealt with. When you have done something to offend someone else, you should take the first step in asking that person to forgive you. This should, however, not become false humility where you constantly ask everyone to forgive you, because you once again are putting yourself in bondage and try-ing to live out religion in an attempt to please.

The third phase in forgiveness is confessing all your sins and wrong-doings to God and asking Him to forgive you of all your sins and cleanse you of all unrighteousness. He is a loving God and will gladly do so; all you need to do is ask.

1.6.2 Ignorance

Lack of knowledge is another mental block to be dealt with in order to unleash your inner passion. The Bible confirms that God's people are destroyed for a lack of knowledge[14] and that you will be set free when you know the Truth.[15]

Make it your mission in life to acquire knowledge in order to overcome this mental block. You should learn the ultimate Truth, that is the Word of God and the principles contained therein, and then begin to live them and put them into practice. You should learn about relationships, about marriage and about sex.

If you do not acquire the necessary knowledge on these related subjects, how do you suppose you are going to overcome the mental block of ignorance in your marriage and sex life?

Overcoming ignorance is a basic step in the right direction of unleashing your inner passion.

1.6.3 Society and culture

Society and culture may be a mental block for you, especially when you allow cultural beliefs and what society expects of you to be the overbearing factor of who you are. Be the person God created you to be and enjoy yourself and your personality as the unique individual God created.

Society should not dictate who you are.

Your culture should not determine who you become.

Enjoy being unique in the midst of your society and culture. Your spouse chose you because of your uniqueness and you should not hide who you are in order for society to 'accept' you; if society does not accept you for who you are, they are in fact not accepting the way God designed you.

Unleashing your inner passion should be a matter between you, your spouse and God. Do not allow society and culture to overburden you and make you feel guilty for being different or maybe wanting to experiment with something not generally acceptable to them. Always determine that what you want to experiment with is aligned with the

Word of God and then discuss it with your spouse, leaving society and culture out of it.

What is much more important than society and culture is being true to yourself and enjoying life and marriage with an unleashed sexual life, making God smile.

If you experienced sexual hurt in your past, it might affect what you will allow in the bedroom, what you will be hesitant about and what you will not even consider. This is something that your spouse must deal with in loving kindness.

Society and cultural rules and regulations do not necessarily provide a valid reason for you not to experiment with something in the bedroom. For example, if you want to experiment with oral sex, but your culture or society frowns upon the practice, rather discuss it with your spouse and together determine the biblical perspective on the subject, then make a decision that is right for you as a couple.

1.7 Sexual hurts

Sexual hurts in a marriage can often arise. It takes just a few encounters of selfish behaviour to understand what I mean. Even if you have never been hurt through sexual misbehaviour, you might want to read this anyway.

It is important for us to be accountable for the bad and the good things in our marriage in order to find a healthy balance with our spouse and God. The moment we recognise a difficulty or something good, we should speak about it for the purpose of working with it. For instance, if when your husband makes love to you, he turns around and falls asleep, you may feel hurt and take a while before you can fall asleep yourself. Immediately say something like: 'I need you to hold me, I need your body warmth against my skin.' Even if he does not want to, he will most probably hold you. Love is stronger than you can imagine. Or your wife might not want to make love. Immediately say something like: 'I want to make love to you and if you don't want to, it's okay, but I really need you right now.' A wise wife will see this as an opportunity to invest in her marriage.

The best way of dealing with sexual hurts is to deal with them immediately and effectively.

So how do you know when you are sexually hurting? There are various degrees of sexual hurt. When small things that are impossible to miss first start to occur, try not to ignore them even though they do not yet affect your marriage. Give this stage a time limit with which you are comfortable, and if things do not change, it is time to deal with the matter by talking about it to your spouse. It might be difficult for you, but you do not have anything to lose and you might even open a door to a higher level of intimacy. Trust opens two doors: setting you free because you are honest and creating intimacy, especially when you are using it to benefit the situation.

There is more than one way to express what you want to say. You can say: 'I need more sex' in a disrespectful manner, while staring at the TV and while your spouse is feeling stressed, or you can say 'I need more sex' over a romantic dinner, whispering in your spouse's ear. Be sensitive in the manner which you express yourself towards your spouse while hurting about something in your sex life.

The next level of intensity of sexual hurting is when you hurt while thinking about the problem. You know there is a problem and you know what it is and it persists even when you speak to your spouse about it. You feel like you are alone in your problem, like there are no answers and you have to accept it the way it is. But the truth is, you do not have to accept the problem and you most certainly are not alone in your problem. Yes, this is a very difficult situation, yes, it is frustrating, but you do have hope, hope we will look at later on.

The last level of intensity of sexual hurt is when you are already packing your bags, you are taking your hurting heart and saving what you can and getting out! You do not care anymore!

This very desperate stage may cause your spouse to pause for a moment and recognise how hard you have been trying to save the relationship, how hard you have searched for the right answers and solutions.

- Having a problem does not mean you have lost the battle;
- Having a problem does not make you weak or less able to carry on with your life;
- It is not a problem that no one else has had before; somewhere there is someone having the same problem or who has had the same problem.
- Problems are conquerable depending on how determined you, together with your spouse, are to overcome them.

It is normal to reach the point where you decide you are leaving. It is okay. We all reach a point where we feel we need time out. Take your bag and sleep ALONE somewhere else to get perspective of the situation and how you are going to move forward. You may wonder how a Christian counsellor can suggest this but it is important for you to be okay first. Before anything else, you matter first to God before your marriage and sexual relationship. Right now, in this phase, that is all you need to focus on.

Many advisors will advise you not to be alone at this point in your relationship. We disagree. The problem is between you and your spouse, not between you, your spouse and a trusted friend.

When you have pulled yourself together, go back to your spouse and discuss how you will solve the problem with a professional to help you. A neutral party does not become part of your marriage or the problem, and afterwards will not remind you of the problem you had. Many couples go to a trusted counsellor or sex therapist for guidance. In the end it is you solving your problem and the counsellor or sex therapist giving you professional guidance.

Having great trusted friends is good. However, friends are supposed to do the friend thing and be friends, not be counsellors or even worse, sex therapists! Friends or family are not trained to help you or your spouse, they are your friends and family. Marriage counsellors and more specifically, Christian sexual therapists, are trained to help you.

Countless couples seek help from their pastor. Again, the pastor is trained to teach you about the Bible and your position in and through the faith, not your sexual relationship. It is very difficult for pastors to cope with the many demands on their time. They really do not have the time or space to deal with personal difficulties. Rather seek to be referred to a marriage counsellor or sexual therapist from your church. They should be geared up to give you professional credited direction. Some churches have counsellors working at the church who are able to assist you.

Do you feel like there is hope already? Do not underestimate your own capacity in solving and overcoming sexual hurt. Also do not underestimate the glue that binds your marriage.

Giving up is a phase of quitting; it is not quitting itself; so is divorce unless both spouses are entering into it by will. When you are entering this phase you have failed to look at the bigger picture God has for you. You are missing the promise of loving your spouse through every high mountain and every low valley until death parts you and you are no longer focussed on your life in eternity. What is the answer? Get back to resolving the problem. You can do it together with your spouse and God. You can make use of the guidance of a good marriage counsellor or sex therapist, praying and working through it step by step.

Sexual hurt is a phase that too shall pass! It is something resolvable. You might not see the solution immediately, neither may your spouse, and the problem might take very long time to resolve; you might even lose hope a few times. But you will resolve it, you will get through it, you will overcome this sexual hurting and you will look back on it some day, knowing you are victorious.

In a healthy sexual relationship you can never make too much love unless it means that you do not have time to spend with God, go to Church or carry on with a normal way of living. It is good to have healthy boundaries.

The sexual hurt between you and your spouse might have to do with a sexual cycle, dormant desires or simple expectations, seeing sex as sin, matters of the past, fear or seeing no love between you, pride, rejection, hate, loneliness, being humiliated, sickness or disability etc. It is not an easy situation to be in and you definitely do not deserve it. You are a God-created human being, you are made to have the best possible sex you can have with your spouse and you have the right to have it.

1.8 Resentment

What is sexual resentment? In easy terms it basically means you have let the problem go too far and too long before taking measures to resolve it. Now bitterness and hatred sneaked in through the back door and more hurts are piled upon your sex life. If by now you have not taken this matter in hand and done something to solve it, you are on the verge of letting your sex life fall apart and you are as guilty as your spouse. It takes two people to rock the sex boat.

You being right about everything and your spouse being guilty is not the point at all. You are part of a destructive situation. You are sleeping apart from each other, not seeing each other in the morning or in the evening, and there is no spiritual, physical or emotional contact between you. What are you going to do to resolve this matter?

Here's how this works. The reality is: is this really the way you want to spend your life? Is this how you see your future? No! It is not what you had in mind when you decided to get married. It is not what you promised your spouse before God. You promised you would be there for them through thick and thin. Right now there is no compromise or compassion, and you have made up your mind to be mad. Your passion has changed to getting back at your spouse for what they have supposedly done!

If you want to resent your spouse for what they have or haven't done to you sexually, you have that choice. You have the choice to be bitter and to despise them for everything they do or try, without even considering whether they are guilty or not.

However, you have forgotten one very small detail in your crafty plan. You have forgotten that you are a blessed child of God. No matter how you look at this, resentment, bitterness and hate has put you in a place of losing what you most deserve, a step closer to receiving pleasure from God through making passionate love to your spouse and your spouse loving you passionately. Does this sound far away from where you are right now? Of course it does, because you are very far away from where you should be.

Whether you are going to let bitterness, resentment and hate kill you emotionally, physically and spiritually is entirely up to you. It is, however, a very lonely place to be and it is a hard life to live. But it is really okay to accept defeat and let resentment, fear, bitterness and hate go! I know it sounds unreasonable but you really can just let it go.

The only way to let it go is to say you are sorry (even if you are not guilty) and mean it. Forgive your spouse for everything they have done to you and make up your mind not to expect anything from them whatsoever (not even to forgive you after you have said you are sorry). This will take some consideration, so please pray about it first. Immediately after forgiving your spouse, pray to God and ask Him to forgive you in the Name of Jesus Christ. Then every morning, pray and ask the Holy Spirit to help you to live a new life in your marriage.

The core problem may still exist but at least now you are able to receive the blessings of God's kingdom while working on a solution to solve the problem.

Try not to become hateful or resentful again, even if the problem persists. You are a person made with love and made able to love unconditionally; anything deviating from this is not good for you.

1.9 Summary

Laying the correct foundations focusses on the pleasure which God intended for a married couple. It is supposed to be just that...pleasure! God gives unconditionally and He gives in abundance, and what He gives, He never takes back. Focus on how to accept this wonderful gift of joy and immense pleasure into your life, discovering how God wants you and your spouse to express your love for each other. Build on what you have right now between you and your spouse, start afresh if you have not done so already by forgiving and moving forward. Accept God's goodness and mercy, and work to achieve sexual pleasure.

Just like embarking on a new adventure, you are about to be blessed when you persist in the goodness and mercy God wants for your sex life, regardless of everything and everyone else. Believe you have it and go for it!

CHAPTER 2

A biblical view on sex

The Bible is the believer's guidance manual and the route map towards living a life to the glory of God. For believers it is of the utmost importance to comply with biblical guidelines to ensure they are in the perfect will of God; the ultimate place to be when you believe in an almighty God and Creator of the whole universe.

Believers see the Bible as the Word of God and it is not difficult to realise why. The Bible is a compilation of 66 books written over a period of about 1 600 years by about 40 different authors, with different cultural backgrounds and education levels, who mostly did not know one another. What makes this so amazing is the central theme of Jesus Christ and the redemption He brought to mankind found throughout the Bible.

What the Bible has to say about sex therefore holds weight to the believer as believers want to live a life pleasing to God in every area of their lives. The message of the Bible may also be of importance to non-believers because it contains certain principles to help people live fulfilled, happy and prosperous lives. The principles of the Bible put into action will work for believers as well as non-believers. The only difference is that believers have a personal relationship with the One who laid down the principles, thus giving them a head start and some valuable 'inside information', guiding them while putting the principles into practice.

Sex is a much talked-about topic in modern-day society; it is portrayed in various forms in the media and it is hard not to take notice of it. When looking at sex in the media ask whether these actions should be lived out within marriage. The best place to search for an answer is from the Creator of the human race Himself and in his Word. So let us have a look at the Bible and what it says about sex and various sexual matters.

It should be clearly stated that the Bible is not a rule book with a whole list of do's and don'ts to spoil your fun. The Bible mentions principles to follow, but all these principles are there to improve the quality of life and ensure happiness. These principles should be seen in context of the biblical passage, though, to ensure its true meaning is seen, understood and applied.

We believe the Bible should always be read in context to lead to the correct biblical interpretation. This basic method prevents people putting their own opinions into Scripture and will encourage people to find the true meaning of the Scripture, regardless of popular opinion or what other denominations believe. Our opinions should be shaped by the Bible and the Bible should not be manipulated to prove our points of view.

Let us start off by saying we are going to look at what the Bible says about sex, but this is how we interpret the Bible on this subject. You may not agree with our interpretation, but just be open enough to read it and take it into consideration. Lastly, just before we embark on this sexual exploration in the Bible, you should realise the Bible might allow a sexual activity and not clearly forbid it, but you do not have to practice it if you are uncomfortable with it or if you dislike the activity or what it entails. So let us start this sexual journey with this in mind.

2.1 Is sexual intercourse a sin?

In some marriages, it might seem as if sex is one of the biggest sins due to absence, but is it? This is exactly what *Between the Covers* is all about; determining what the Bible says about sex so that you can unleash your inner sexual passion.

God created humans in his own image as male and female, according to Genesis 1:27, and in Genesis 1:28 He commands them to have sex and to multiply and reproduce. The Bible clearly states here God invented and created sex and even told men and women to have sex.

Is sexual intercourse thus a sin? Definitely not! God invented sex, but as the inventor of sex He also has certain principles to help you enjoy it to the full and use it as He originally intended. If someone invented something, he or she is the best person to ask how it is supposed to work or to provide the owner's manual on how it is supposed to work. The same is true when it comes to sex. God invented it and therefore He also gave his Word, the Bible, as the owner's manual to help humans implement it in the correct way to avoid unnecessary hurt and pain. God's plan for sex is found summarised in one verse of the Bible.

'And the man and his wife were both naked and were not embarrassed *or* ashamed in each other's presence.'[16] From this verse it is evident these people were comfortable being naked with each other because they knew God gave them permission and even commanded them to have sex. They knew and lived out God's plan for sex and they were comfortable with that.

In this Scripture three very important principles are found about what God's original plan regarding sex was supposed to be. Firstly, we see that God created a man and a woman and told them to have sex. God's original plan was thus for sex to be used in a heterosexual relationship. Secondly, it is seen that the man and his wife were naked, in other words, sex was not just meant to be used in any heterosexual relationship, but within a heterosexual marriage. Thirdly, sex was meant to be used in a heterosexual marriage between one man and one woman.

Obviously this is not the popular view in the world and media today, but it is the biblical view and, as said previously, we need to readjust our lives to align ourselves with the Bible.

In Leviticus 18 a whole list is given of restrictions on sexual intercourse, but when looking at this list it is common sense to see that the result of such sex will only lead to unnecessary heartache, hurt and pain. When looking at these God-given rules, they forbid having sexual intercourse with family so it is not difficult to comprehend what the result will be when these rules are not adhered to. The sad part of reading this Scripture is if you look at modern-day TV soap-operas it is as if the directors took this Scripture and everything God forbids and wrote it into the storyline, because most soap-operas are basically a portrayal of everything God clearly forbids in these verses.

In the Ten Commandments God clearly forbids adultery[17] as well as coveting your neighbour's spouse.[18] There are clearly situations where sexual intercourse is classified as sin by God Himself and is strictly forbidden, not because God wants to spoil your fun, but because He wants to protect you from unnecessary hurt and pain. Sexual intercourse with your spouse inside the confines of marriage is not sin, however, but what about various sexual activities? Numerous sexual activities are represented in the media, but are they all permissible with your spouse?

We are about to enter a territory of sexuality where very few Christians dare to even peek, so prepare yourself for the time has come to call a sexual activity by its name and see what the Bible has to say about it. Before we do, however, you should realise from the beginning the Bible might not have anything to say about a certain subject and in those cases the activity will be viewed from a point of logic, experience and morality. You should also prepare yourself to hear the truth about what the Bible says and not be heavy laden by needless beliefs put on you by culture, tradition and religion.

The biblical way is based on freedom because Jesus Christ took our sin upon Himself and He has set us free from having to live our lives with a rule book in one hand and fear of committing a terrible sin in the other. You are to live your life based on the freedom you find in Him and accordingly, you should live and enjoy your Christian marriage. You should unleash your inner passion in your marriage to enjoy your sexuality and live as a sexually fulfilled spouse.

2.2 What happens in the spiritual realm when you have sex?

To fully understand what happens in the spiritual realm when two people are having sex, it should first be determined who we are as Christian believers. The Bible says a person who is united to the Lord becomes one spirit with Him.[19] Christians are united with the Lord because of accepting the sacrifice Jesus Christ made for them on the cross and therefore every Christian becomes one spirit with Him. This whole line of thought continues:

'Do you not know that your body is the temple (the very sanctuary) of the Holy Spirit Who lives within you, Whom you have received [as a Gift] from God? You are not your own. You were bought with a price [purchased with a preciousness and paid for, made His own]. So then, honor God *and* bring glory to Him in your body.'[20] It is made clear by the Bible that Christians are directly connected to God in the spiritual realm. When looking at sexuality in this light it is clear that when you have sex with someone, you are involving God in that action since He is part of you.

Fully understanding this will make you understand why the Bible says believers should not be unequally yoked with non-believers[21] meaning Christians should not get married to non-believers. Once again, it is not to spoil your fun. It is all about Christians being one with God, and being sexually involved with a non-believer defiles God's character of purity since light and darkness cannot become one. In the Bible it is stated that sexual intercourse causes two people to become one flesh[22] and even confirmed in the New Testament which states that when a man joins himself to a prostitute, he becomes one body with her.[23] It is also said that sexual immorality is sin against his body while all other sin takes place outside the body.[24]

Looking at all these Scriptures makes you realise that sexual intercourse is not just an instinct to fulfil lusty bodily desires; sex is a spiritual matter involving both partners as well as God. When sexual intercourse takes place, both partners are spiritually linked to each other as well as with God. During sexual intercourse the partners literally become one in body. Sexual partners can even experience this spiritual attachment when they begin to 'read each other's thoughts'.

Sex is much more than just activities to kill time or to fulfil your desires. Sexual intercourse is the mingling together of two people for them to truly become one in the spiritual realm. It is more than a physical act, it is a total intertwining of two people's spirits, souls and bodies in the presence of the Almighty God.

Understanding what happens in the spiritual realm when people have sex makes the whole matter of adultery and extramarital sex much more complicated than just some pleasure on the side. What happens in the spiritual realm during extramarital sex is actually the connection of a third person, along with this person's past sexual partners, to your marriage and descendents.

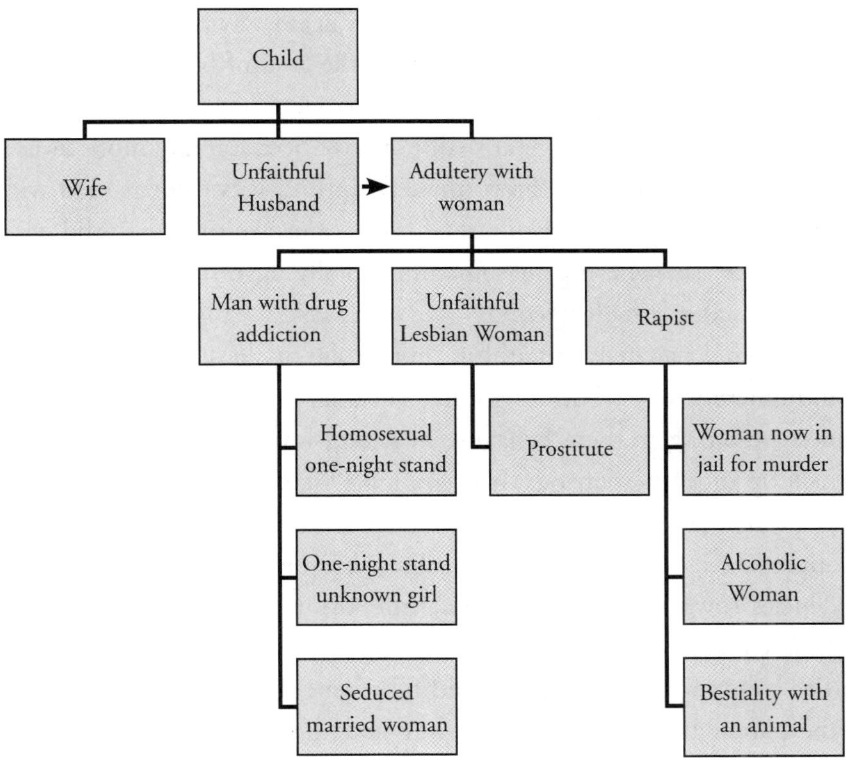

In this diagram it is seen when a spouse gets involved in extramarital sex, a union does not only take place between the unfaithful spouse and the third party, but this third person with her background is also brought into the marriage. In the spiritual realm they are all being attached, resulting in a child being born into the marriage with negative tendencies towards sexual sin, addiction, seduction, prostitution, rape, alcoholism and so forth. Does this mean the child will definitely struggle with these things? Absolutely not! What might happen is more of a tendency for the child towards it. However, the Bible clearly says that children will not be punished for their parents' sin and mistakes[25] so it is not a given that the child will battle with these things.

Generational curses may exist and affect a person's life, but generational curses cannot be seen as a law that the child will definitely suffer from the things brought into the family by the unfaithful parent. The Bible is clear about this when it states:

'The Word of the Lord came to me again, saying, what do you mean by using this proverb concerning the land of Israel, The fathers have eaten sour grapes, and the children's teeth are set on edge? As I live, says the Lord God, you shall not have occasion any more to use this proverb in Israel.'[26] From these Scriptures it is evident God will not allow the child to be punished for the mistake the unfaithful parent made, so believing in something totally against what the Bible frankly states is foolishness.

When a parent is unfaithful, though, he or she lives out their sin in numerous ways. They might live out their guilt, shame and foolishness, resulting in them behaving in wrong ways and the child might pick up on this behaviour. It is common knowledge that children do what their parents do and not what they say. Based on this behavioural approach, it is not difficult to realise why the child might have tendencies towards the sins brought into the family by the unfaithful parent and it has nothing to do with so-called generational curses. The child might mirror the unfaithful parent's behaviour due to seeing the parent behave in a certain way and the child picks up on the behaviour. Blaming so-called generational curses for a child's behaviour is a cop-out and just a way for the parent to shift blame for his or her own sinful unfaithfulness and not own up to the mistakes made and the sins committed.

These same Scriptures state parents will be punished for their own sins so for the person who had extramarital sex, there will surely be consequences; inability to communicate with God, guilt, shame, perversity, lack of respect from the children and spouse, and much more. It may also cause the child to rebel and actually act out the exact same behaviour of the parent, therefore the reason there might be an increased tendency in the spiritual realm towards these actions. We can see that the child is not spiritually affected in the form of a generational curse by the unfaithful parent's sinful behaviour, but the child might be behaviourally affected, thus acting out in rebellion what has been observed in the parent's life.

The diagram shows one matter very clearly, namely the unfaithful spouse becoming one in adultery with another person, but also with all previous sexual partners of that person. The unfaithful husband in the diagram is therefore the one who will in the spiritual realm be directly influenced by the adulterating woman's previous sexual partner's sin. The unfaithful husband will struggle with and be tempted with thoughts of and matters like sexual sin, addiction, prostitution, homosexuality, casual sex, alcoholism and so forth. Physically the unfaithful husband did not only have sex with the woman, but actually with all her previous sexual partners as well, because if one of them had a sexually transmitted disease, he might get it as well. This is why an unfaithful spouse usually struggles with a need for more sexual sin.

The spouse of the unfaithful partner will also be directly influenced by the sin of her husband, but not in the sense of being connected with the 'other woman's' previous sexual partners. The wife did not sin and will not experience the same negative tendencies although she and her husband are already one. What the wife will experience is an emotional distance with her husband and their marriage might develop problems due to the husband becoming more and more dissatisfied with the marriage and sex with his wife. The unfaithful husband's actions and sin influence his marriage, but his sin is not carried over to his wife and the wife will not be punished for the husband's wrongdoings.

What should you do if you had feet of clay, fell for temptation and were involved in an extramarital affair? Two Scriptures provide us with an answer:

'The soul that sins, it [is the one that] shall die. The son shall not bear and be punished for the iniquity of the father, neither shall the father bear and be punished for the iniquity of the son; the righteousness of the righteous shall be upon him only, and the wickedness of the wicked shall be upon the wicked only. But if the wicked man turns from all his sins that he has committed and keeps all My statutes and does that which is lawful and right, he shall surely live; he shall not die.'[27]

The second Scripture is where Jesus personally answered a woman who was caught in adultery and His response was the following:

'She answered, 'No one, Lord!' And Jesus said, 'I do not condemn you either. Go on your way and from now on sin no more.'"[28]

Jesus came to earth for people to have an abundant and enjoyable life[29] and therefore He only wants the best for everyone. The best includes a happy marriage and family life. When a spouse makes the mistake of falling into an extramarital affair and committing adultery, it will only lead to unhappiness and spiritual death of the involved person and negative tendencies hanging over the family. This is definitely not what Jesus wants for us.

You might be the one who committed adultery and brought bad vibes and negative tendencies into your family. We have good news for you; Jesus wants to set you free. You do not have to live with this guilt and shame any longer. What you need to do is to confess your sin, the adultery, openly to God. You should then accept His forgiveness and in the process forgive yourself for falling into temptation.

The next step is to recommit your life to God and make Jesus the Lord of your whole life. Then you should ask God to set you free from sexual sin and cleanse you of all unrighteousness. You will soon realise that if you cannot do this on your own, it might be a good idea to visit a minister of the Gospel, a Christian counsellor or a Christian leader you can trust and who knows how to pray effectively. Confessing your sin to God in this person's presence and allowing the person to pray a prayer of deliverance from the sexual sin over you not only makes the prayer very effective, it also sets you up for success because you now have someone to be accountable to regarding your sexual purity in the future.

Maybe you are the person who found out your spouse committed adultery and need some clarity on what to do. Your biggest challenge, but yet the most important part of moving forward, is to forgive your spouse. With God's help this is possible and after you have truly forgiven, you are in the best position to decide what your options are for the future and for your marriage. You have every right to want a divorce, but is it really the best option for you? You are the only one able to answer that question, but do not make a decision based on emotional hurt that you might regret later on. Rather deal with what happened and forgive your spouse in order for you to make the correct decision based from an emotionally sound perspective. Remember, forgiveness is not for your spouse, it is for you. You have to release the pain, the hurt and the violation of your world in order for you not to be bound by the past, but rather to enter the future without baggage. Only then will you be in a position to make a sound decision about your future and the future of your marriage.

2.3 Sexual activities

Sex is much more than only sexual penetration during intercourse; it may involve many sexual activities and we will now discuss them and what the Bible's point of view is on these activities. It should be clearly noted these sexual activities are looked at from the perspective of the sexual partners being spouses in a Christian heterosexual marriage.

Within the boundaries of marriage you should be able to communicate openly with your spouse and have such a wonderfully close relationship with each other that you can allow yourselves to truly explore your sexuality. A good rule of thumb regarding sexuality is to allow anything in the bedroom with your spouse as long as there is no direct biblical guideline prohibiting it and you are both comfortable with it. If one of you are uncomfortable with a sexual activity, even though it might not be biblically ruled out, rather do not get involved with it due to your love for your spouse and always keeping your spouse's comfort above your own. On the other hand, do not inhibit your spouse from sexual exploration with you just because of beliefs you have about a certain activity based on what others told you or what you have heard from others. Be open enough to explore your and your spouse's sexuality together.

Just before we explore some sexual activities and see what the Bible has to say, let us just spend some time looking at three Scriptures to guide you while browsing through some of the sexual activities that follow. Keep these Scriptures in mind when considering any sexual activity.

'Everything is permissible (allowable and lawful) for me; but not all things are helpful (good for me to do, expedient and profitable when considered with other things). Everything is lawful for me, but I will not become the slave of anything *or* be brought under its power.'[30] While exploring some sexual activities within your marriage, always keep in mind that although something might be allowable to you, it might not be beneficial for you or your marital relationship and you should never get involved in any sexual activity causing you to be enslaved to it.

'This is in keeping with my own eager desire *and* persistent expectation *and* hope, that I shall not disgrace myself *nor* be put to shame in anything; but that with the utmost freedom of speech *and* unfailing courage, now as always heretofore, Christ (the Messiah) will be magnified *and* get glory *and* praise in this body of mine *and* be boldly exalted in my person, whether through (by) life or through (by) death.'[31] Whatever sexual activity you want to explore, you should always magnify God through the activity and never do anything causing you or your spouse to be put to shame or be degraded.

'So any person who knows what is right to do but does not do it, to him it is sin.'[32] It is evident from this Scripture that even though the Bible might not prohibit a certain sexual activity, but you believe it is not right to do it, rather stay clear from it, because for you it will be sin. When you allow the Holy Spirit to lead you and guide you through all the decisions you take on a daily basis, you can be sure of being in God's perfect will for you.

Something might be wrong for you to do, but not necessarily for others. To give you an example, to someone it might be wrong to use alcohol because God wants the person to abstain from it due to a certain calling on his or her life, so if this person uses alcohol it is wrong and a sin for him or her. Does this mean the use of alcohol is a sin for everyone? No, Jesus Himself drank wine when He was on the earth, but for the person who received a specific instruction from God to abstain from alcohol it will be a sin if the instruction is ignored. The same is true when it comes to sexual activities; although the Bible may not prohibit it, you might feel in your heart God is telling you not to get involved in it and then you should stay clear of it, but at the same time not judging others who are practising it.

Everything you do should be for the glory of God and when you have sex with your spouse in marriage, it should be to make God smile. When you get involved in sexual activities with your spouse it should still be for the glorification of God and for the enjoyment of both of you.

So having said all of this as a foundation, let us continue our journey through the Bible in our search to determine the biblical view on sexuality. Keep in mind, when looking at the following sexual activities, that they can be used within marriage as foreplay or to reach orgasm, and a distinction will have to be made between these two categories.

2.3.1 Sexual fantasy

Sexual fantasy is imagining sexual acts and thinking sexual thoughts about someone.

'You have heard that it was said, you shall not commit adultery. But I say to you that everyone who so much as looks at a woman with evil desire for her has already committed adultery with her in his heart.'[33]

Within this short Scripture the whole matter of sexual fantasy has been dealt with unambiguously. Sexual fantasy within marriage has its place when you are having fantasies about your spouse, but when you have sexual fantasies about anyone other than your spouse, you are sinning and this is not allowed in a believer's marriage. Jesus said this is just as bad as adultery and it may eventually cause you to become dissatisfied with your spouse. If you become unhappy with your sex life, it may even reach the point where you are no longer sexually satisfied if there is no sexual fantasy involved.

Sexual fantasies about your spouse during the day, however, are preparing you for the sexual intimacy to follow and are a form of foreplay. When approached as such they will assist in you being sexually prepared to offer your spouse deserved intimacy when you are together. In a way this may even prepare both spouses to be ready for sex when they are together and reduce the need for foreplay into a desire for foreplay.

2.3.2 Manual sex

Manual sex is when you stimulate your spouse's genitals either as foreplay or to bring about orgasm. Manual sex can be done as a mutual act where your spouse will do the same for you as you stimulate your spouse's genitals or as a marital act of love by helping to relieve your partner's sexual tension since you are not in the mood to have sex.

Manual sex differentiates from masturbation in that manual sex is when your partner stimulates your genitals and in masturbation you stimulate your own genitals. What does the Bible say about manual sex?

The Bible does not directly talk about manual sex, but as seen in 1 Corinthians 7:5 you should not refuse your spouse sex and this is a sexual method to be used when sexual intercourse is not desired or possible for some or other reason. Manual sex is also an alternative to usual sexual intercourse and another way you may unleash your inner sexual passion or explore some new avenues of sexuality with your spouse.

2.3.3 Outer sex

Another way to help relieve your spouse's sexual tension, and even be stimulating for you too, is outer sex. Outer sex is used during foreplay or to reach orgasm for one or both spouses and it is done without actual vaginal, oral or anal penetration. Two methods for outer sex are firstly for the spouses to rub their bodies and genitals against each other (even while clothed) and secondly to properly lubricate the penis and then insert it between the wife's thighs, buttocks, breasts or feet.

The Bible has nothing to say about outer sex. As long as it happens between two married spouses, there is nothing wrong with it as long as both partners feel comfortable with it.

2.3.4 Oral sex

Oral sex is the stimulation of your spouse's genitals with your mouth and tongue as part of foreplay or to bring about orgasm. Oral sex is for mutual pleasure or a way of pleasing your partner sexually.

The Bible does not prohibit oral sex and it is a natural part of foreplay, but may also be used to help a spouse reach orgasm.

Many people may not like the idea of putting their mouths close to or on their spouse's genitals and therefore avoid oral sex. Two points to make here are firstly, that oral sex is a very stimulating part of foreplay or sex and when practiced, many spouses find it highly erotic and enjoyable. The second point is that when you or your spouse find oral sex offensive, you should maybe spend some time determining why. Maybe the perception is based on your cultural background, your upbringing or sexual abuse in your past.

The question is necessary because your spouse might long for oral sex and you do not, but maybe there is a valid reason for your offence that might be effectively dealt with so that you to overcome it. It might be worth your while to spend some time determining why you feel the way you do so you may understand yourself better and enlighten your spouse accordingly, and then you may together discuss the appropriate way forward for the two of you.

2.3.5 Sex during menstruation

'Also you shall not have intercourse with a woman during her [menstrual period or similar] uncleanness.'[34] The Bible clearly says to avoid sexual intercourse during menstruation, but looking at this Scripture in context it also says a woman who menstruates should totally separate herself from her family since she and even the furniture she sits on is unclean and should not be touched.[35] These Scriptures say that when a woman menstruates, her husband should not have sex with her or even sleep on the same bed, sit next to her on the coach, touch her or be near her.

What does this mean? The regulations about menstruation were not so much about sex during menstruation as for two main reasons; firstly for sanitary reasons due to the Israelites living in the desert and therefore not having proper access to hygienic cleaning methods, and secondly due to living under the Old Covenant. It should be remembered in the Old Testament people were not allowed to touch blood, because then they would be unclean in the eyes of God and therefore could not come close to the tabernacle, as seen in the same Scripture.

'Thus you shall separate the Israelites from their uncleanness, lest they die in their uncleanness by defiling My tabernacle that is in the midst of them.'[36]

When Jesus Christ came to the earth and died on the cross for all the sins of mankind, His blood was shed and it broke the Old Covenant and initiated the New Covenant. This means being in contact with blood no longer defiles people since the Church is no longer under the law, but under the freedom of the New Covenant, where Jesus' blood took care of all uncleanness. Therefore people come into God's presence because of the sacrifice of Jesus[37] and not because of being 'clean' from not touching blood and bodily fluids.

Does this mean sex during menstruation is allowed? Biblically it is not forbidden when reading every applicable Scripture in its full context, but it is a matter of preference between the spouses. Some couples might not like the idea of having sex when there is blood around and sexual penetration is therefore avoided, but they may make use of alternative sex, like outer sex, during the time of menstruation.

Medically there are different opinions about sex during menstruation; one stream of medical practitioners encourage it and believe orgasm will release endorphins in the bloodstream, reducing pain during menstruation, but on the other side there is a medical view of increased blood flow and therefore sex during menstruation is discouraged. Whatever your opinion, just know the Bible does not clearly forbid sex during menstruation and whether you like or dislike the idea is based on you and your spouse's personal opinion. Remember that there are alternatives available for sex during menstruation which do not involve actual sexual penetration. There is thus no reason to totally avoid your wife during her time of menstruation.

2.3.6 Birth control

The Bible does not clearly prohibit or approve birth control, so once again it is a matter each married couple should decide for themselves. Birth control means taking certain products or medication to prevent pregnancies. There are certain points to consider, though, and the first one is the example of Onan in Genesis 38:8-10. The story of Onan mentions a certain method of birth control, but it should be clearly stated God was not unhappy about the birth control practiced in this Scripture, but about the disregard for the very important custom of the day.

It should also be mentioned how God created people and commanded them to multiply and procreate in Genesis 1:26-28, so why does the Bible not clearly answer the question about birth control? God created people in His own image according to this Scripture, meaning each person has free will and the ability to make their own decisions. God gave people this ability and He entrusted the whole earth to them, including the responsibility of leading their own lives and making decisions for their families. Based on this point of view, a Scripture to be looked at is:

'Do not refuse *and* deprive *and* defraud each other [of your due marital rights], except perhaps by mutual consent for a time, so that you may devote yourselves unhindered to prayer. But afterwards resume marital relations, lest Satan tempt you [to sin] through your lack of restraint of sexual desire.'[38]

This Scripture does not talk about birth control as such, but an important principle can be seen here. God gave married couples the ability to decide by mutual agreement to abstain from sex for a limited period to devote themselves to prayer. It therefore stands to reason when a married couple prayerfully make a decision together not to have any more children and then use birth control, God will not stand in their way. The decision to use birth control is one of the most loving decisions any couple can take to ensure they are able to provide in the best possible ways for their children without putting unnecessary economic strain on themselves and their children.

What should be understood is the Bible's clear instruction not to commit murder.[39] It is believed when the husband's sperm connects with the wife's ovum, conception takes place and then a new life is formed in that very instance. Any method for birth control should consequently prevent conception rather than eliminate the newly formed life after it has been created.

Various forms of birth control exist of which the most common is probably the use of male or female condoms. The more radical approaches involve a full or partial hysterectomy for the wife or a vasectomy for the husband. We mention this specifically because of the big decisions involved in permanent sterilisation.

A hysterectomy is usually a big operation and may have severe consequences. A partial hysterectomy is often more desirable because only the womb is removed, thus leaving all the other female organs so the woman can still produce her own hormones; this is not the case in a full hysterectomy. The pros and cons of a hysterectomy should be thoroughly discussed with a gynaecologist before embarking on that route. That being said, after a partial or full hysterectomy women may still enjoy a healthy sex life.

A vasectomy is a much smaller operation with less risk involved. Whatever route is taken, sex afterwards is in general very exciting and without the risk and fear of unwanted pregnancy.

2.3.7 Interracial sex

What does the Bible say about sex between spouses of different races? Well, the answer is easy; nothing. The Bible does not mention sex between partners of different races. What the Bible does mention is the fact of not making an issue of different races and seeing people of all races as equals.

'[No one] for there is no distinction between Jew and Greek. The same Lord is Lord over all [of us] and He generously bestows His riches upon all who call upon Him [in faith].'[40] It is said without doubt God does not discriminate against anyone and especially not based on the colour of their skin. God sees all people as equals so the matter of interracial marriages and sex between spouses of different races is not even a relevant matter. God gives every person a free will to choose whom he or she will marry and it is not based on the colour of their skins. What the Bible does warn against is for Christians to get involved with unbelievers.

'Do not be unequally yoked with unbelievers [do not make mismated alliances with them or come under a different yoke with them, inconsistent with your faith]...'[41] The Bible prohibits marriages and sex between believer and non-believers, but this does not have anything to do with race. The only consideration when people of different races are married is what the influence of their different cultural backgrounds will be on their marriage, sex lives and children.

2.3.8 Sex toys

Sex toys are devices used by a couple during foreplay or to bring about orgasm and include things like dildos (penis substitute), vibrators (vibrating penis substitutes), flavoured lubrication, vagina moulds (vagina substitute) and many more.

Sex toys are not mentioned in the Bible. There is no moral objection or biblical principle putting a stop to the use of sex toys for married couples. These toys may be very beneficial for variety in foreplay or may be used to help a spouse who finds it difficult to climax to reach orgasm. They may also be of great value when normal sex is not possible, for example, when a wife has an infection or when a husband suffers from impotence.

When using sex toys it should be remembered to treat your spouse with respect and to not shame him or her in any way. Care should also be taken when sex toys are used not to cause injury to your spouse, but to be gentle and comply with the instructions of the specific toy.

2.3.9 Fetish

A fetish is an excessive focus on something to the point where sex is impossible without it or without fantasising about it. Fetishes include various objects, body parts or activities. Before looking at a few sexual fetishes you should realise the Bible plainly states you should not become the slave of anything or be brought under its power[42] and a fetish violates this biblical principle, so a fetish is directly against what the Bible teaches. A fetish also has the ability to change into something, that causes a spouse to feel degraded and worthless; also a principle against the norm of the Bible since people are valuable in the eyes of God.

If you have a fetish towards something you should determine where it comes from and deal with it appropriately since a fetish usually is developed during childhood based on a feeling of incompetence, the inability to perform or as a result of sexual molestation or abuse.

When looking at the following list of some familiar sexual fetishes, please remember there is a big difference between a fetish and a preference. Some people might prefer something, but it is not compulsory and then it is not seen as a fetish.

Fetish objects include things like spandex, leather, high heels, red clothing and certain lingerie.

Fetish body parts include specific hair colour or eye colour, certain sized breasts, buttocks, specific colour pubic hair or the lack of pubic hair and an excessive fascination with feet.

Fetish activities include various things, for example:

- BDSM (Bondage, Domination, Sadomasochism) – dominating your spouse or being dominated by your spouse to be sexually aroused
- Spanking – spanking your spouse or being spanked in order to be sexually aroused
- Watersport – urinating on your spouse and/or have your spouse urinate on you in order to be sexually aroused

These are just a few examples and there are many more possible fetishes and some of them are pretty weird and disgusting. Just about anything can change into a fetish and when you have a fetish you should determine where it comes from, why you feel the need for it and why you are unable to be sexually aroused without this specific object, body part or activity. Your marital sex life will be tremendously enhanced if you are able to overcome the fetish restraining you.

2.4 Summary

Sex in marriage is not about rules and regulations; it is about fully enjoying your spouse and your spouse's body while expressing your love for your spouse physically and sexually. Sex should never be a chore; it should be the most exciting part of your day and of your time with your spouse. Never make sex about rules and regulations, rather make it about joint fun.

If you feel as if sex has become a chore and an activity you try to avoid at all costs, you should determine the reason for that and deal with it appropriately. As we have seen in this chapter, the Bible is clear about God wanting spouses to enjoy sex and each other, and that a spouse should not refuse sex. You may be the spouse never wanting to have sex or refusing your spouse sex all the time and if it is you, God says you are out of his will and you should return to his perfect will for your marriage and life.

There are various sexual activities married couples may get involved in, but whatever sexual activities are pursued or experimented with, always keep your spouse's comfort and pleasure in mind and above your own. You should treat your spouse with respect, regardless of what sexual activities you get involved in and the best rule of thumb is to never do anything you and your spouse do not agree upon. Sex is supposed to be a selfless act, so always put your spouse's needs and wants above your own, as the Bible commands when it says husbands and wives should submit to each and be subject to one another out of reverence for Christ.[43]

A few sexual activities are undoubtedly prohibited by the Bible and as a Christian couple you should avoid them. The activities not clearly prohibited by the Bible may be experimented with if both you and your spouse are comfortable with them and not repelled by anything regarding them. As you embark on this experimentation just remember to do everything with love and respect. On the other hand also, do not be afraid to try out new sexual activities and positions, but be adventurous enough to go with your spouse on a journey of sexual exploration.

Threesomes, homosexuality and lesbianism have not been looked at in this chapter because it is not in the scope of this book to look at all these matters in detail. What should be stressed is that spouses should be faithful to each other and they should not bring a third person of any gender into the marriage, and that includes threesomes, homosexual or lesbian contact. The Christian marriage is a devoted relationship between one man and one woman who should be loyal to each other and be willing to help each other to be sexually fulfilled within the marriage.

Unleashing your inner passion is a process of experimentation and you should not hold back; rather enjoy every moment with your spouse and do not be prudish, but be brave enough to embark on this journey with a smile and you will soon have a much bigger smile on your face while making your spouse smile like never before!

Let us continue our journey toward unleashing the sexual passion hidden inside you by looking in the next chapter at certain traumas and negative effects you might have experienced in the past, preventing you from fully unleashing your inner passion.

These inhibitions should be faced head-on and not side-stepped so that you are not chained to the past. Hurts, pains, traumas and historical negative experiences are a way of holding onto the past, leading to you being incapable of fully giving yourself to your spouse. Effectively dealing with these past negative sexual effects will help you to be willing and wanting to unleash your inner passion to ensure a happy marriage and make your spouse the happiest married person you possibly can.

CHAPTER 3

You are a sexual being

God created you as a sexual being, and embracing your sexuality is the process of unleashing the passion hidden inside you, within the safe boundaries of marriage.

A question you may ask is why your sexual passion is hidden?

It may be due to sexual trauma you experienced earlier on in your life. It may also be a matter of fear; fear of letting go and enjoying your sexuality. The sexual passion may be hidden because of past sexual experiences and, as a result, you are now experiencing guilt. You may be hiding your sexual passion deep inside because of a lack of knowledge regarding your own and your spouse's sexuality and body.

As a sexual being your sexuality is part of you and instead of avoiding or ignoring it, you should embrace it and actively discover it. In this way you facilitate the unleashing of your inner sexual passion.

You may feel uncomfortable about this process of unleashing your inner passion and that is totally understandable. Your past experiences influence the way you feel about sex, but you should be open enough to consider change, especially when it is a change for the better.

Something you should be aware of is the possibility that your present beliefs, attitudes and paradigms about sexuality are totally inappropriate within your marriage and they may actually be hurting your spouse and your marriage. Anything hurting your marriage should be faced and dealt with in order for it to be the marriage God intended it to be.

Sex in marriage should never be seen as a household chore, but rather a time of relaxation, fun and enjoyment you share with your spouse. If you are not enjoying sex, it is your responsibility to do something about it; handle it appropriately so that you may overcome whatever it is holding you back from sexual fulfilment in your marriage. If you are not enjoying sex, then your spouse is also not enjoying it, because marital sexual fulfilment is a two-way process. Readjust your sexuality to ensure sexual fulfilment in your marriage, not only for yourself but for your spouse as well.

Starting this journey of sexual discovery and healing of negative past influences is a process of love; love for God, yourself and your spouse. Being willing to do what it takes to ensure sexual fulfilment in your marriage is a selfless act of love and a sure sign of your commitment to make a success of your marriage.

The journey of unleashing your inner passion continues here by discovering your sexual organs and those of your spouse to become aware of how your bodies were designed to function. Then we will look at some of the past experiences that may influence your sexual fulfilment in your marriage, while looking at some practical steps on how to overcome these difficulties.

3.1 Discovering the genitals

Discovering your genitals and those of your spouse is not a difficult and daunting task, but rather an exciting expedition to be embarked on by everyone. It is up to you to discover your own genitals and know how they work, what you like and what you dislike so you are able to inform your spouse as well.

Understanding the genitals is the first step towards mutual pleasure and an amazing sex life, so if you want to enjoy truly fulfilling sex, get to know your own body and then spend time getting to know your spouse's body. Knowing how the genitals function will give you the advantage of turning your mediocre sex life into a truly fulfilling sexual experience.

Genitals are the sexual body parts that distinguish males and females from one other.

A complete physiological explanation of the genitals is not intended, but rather an overview of the different parts to clearly indicate their location, which you can recall during sexual intercourse to ensure ultimate fulfilment and technique.

3.1.1 Male genitals

The male genitals are very prominent and situated outside the body, except for the prostate gland which is located inside. The scrotum is situated underneath the penis and contains the testicles. The penis consists of the shaft and the very sensitive part, the glans, normally covered with the foreskin if a man is not circumcised.

Circumcision is the process where the foreskin is removed to leave the glans penis uncovered; it may be done for cultural, religious or hygienic reasons. A circumcised glans penis may be a little bit less sensitive, but with it may come the added advantage of the man being able to withhold ejaculation longer; however, this is not always the case and a lot has to do with sexual experience and practise.

During sexual excitement the penis becomes erect and glands secrete a fluid to lubricate the urethra for easy passage of the semen during ejaculation. This lubricating fluid may be secreted from the penis even before the man reaches orgasm and since it may already contain sperm, there is the possibility of this fluid causing pregnancy, even though orgasm has not been reached. The coitus interruptus contraceptive method, i.e. withdrawing the penis from the vagina just before orgasm, is therefore not a very reliable method of contraception and pregnancy may still occur even though the semenal ejaculation of orgasm has not taken place.

3.1.2 Female genitals

The breasts are not usually seen as part of the female genitals, but we believe they are as they are the first point of sexual contact between husband and wife. Because breasts are an obvious part of the female figure, they are often a huge turn-on for men looking at women. Some men are attracted to small breasts while others prefer larger ones, and this fascination causes many women to actually surgically enlarge or reduce their breast sizes.

Sexual excitement causes the nipples to enlarge and get harder while the areolas, the darker part of the breasts surrounding the nipple, contracts. This is exactly the same effect cold weather has on the breasts. The areola changes structure after the birth of a child, changing from smooth to bumpier while the breasts lose firmness as the women gets older. But while the breasts change, they are still the women's outer portrayal of her sexuality.

The vulva is the external female genital. The female reproductive system is rather complicated, consisting of glands, tubes, a uterus and ovaries, all necessary for reproduction and for the menstrual cycle to function effectively. The whole process of menstruation and reproduction falls outside the scope of *Between the Covers* so we will have a look at the vulva, which is directly related to the process of sexual intercourse and foreplay.

The clitoris is the small, sensitive part of the female genitals at the anterior end of the vulva. It also consists of a shaft moving downward into the glans clitoris, just like the penis in the man. The clitoris is sometimes called the 'female penis'. Stimulating the clitoris directly or indirectly is very arousing for women and it leads to lubricating fluid being released inside the vagina and eventually to orgasm.

The labia are the lips covering the vagina. The labia majora are the outer lips and just inside them are the labia minora or the small lips. The labia minora are much more sensitive than the labia majora and when women get aroused and ready for penetration, their labia minora increases in size.

The vagina, which is the passageway from the vaginal opening to the cervix and the uterus, is the canal where the penis is inserted during sexual intercouse. The vaginal opening has many nerves and is very sensitive and arousing when stimulated. Virgins usually have a membrane, the hymen, at the vaginal opening until it is broken with first penetration. Virgins usually have a hymen, because it can be physically torn from activities like riding a bicycle, horseback riding and so forth without sexual intercourse, but just because it is torn physically does not take away from the girl still being seen as a virgin.

3.2 Sexual belief

The sexual being that you are comes from not only your gender but also your sexual beliefs. What you believe about sex and sexuality has a major influence on your life and marriage. Your sexual beliefs have been formed throughout your whole life and influence your marriage and sexuality consciously or subconsciously.

The Bible says: 'Guard your heart above all else, for it determines the course of your life.'[44] What is in your heart, your very inner being, is what you truly believe and cherish. It is your core belief about sexuality that determines how you perceive sex and how you will have sex. What you believe about sex in your heart is how you will act towards sex in your marriage.

Sexual beliefs are the very core of what determines your sexual behaviour. If you believe sex is dirty and something to be ashamed of, you will hide your inner passion and avoid sex as far as possible. If you believe sex is a gift from God and something to enjoy, you will unleash your inner passion, be adventurous in your marriage and have a fulfilling sex life.

Your view on sexuality determines your sexual behaviour and it might even be happening without you even realising it. If you have believed in something for an extended period of time, you will become so used to it that you may not even realise it leads to destructive behaviour.

Where do your beliefs about sexuality come from?

Were they formed during your formative years? Were they shaped due to negative things your parents said about sexuality? Were they outlined by peers portraying fornication as the norm or by television representing it as a conquest to have sex with as many people as possible? Maybe your sexual beliefs came from religious authority figures making you feel guilty about sex to prevent you from having sex?

Wherever your sexual beliefs come from, you should realise your past has influenced what you believe about sex at this moment in your life. If you grew up feeling guilty about sex, you will still be living it out in your marriage and suppressing your inner passion. The result will be an unfulfilled sex life for you and a very boring sex life for your spouse.

You owe it to yourself and to your spouse to effectively deal with all the negative sexual beliefs you are carrying around inside you. It is not healthy having negative sexual beliefs based on your past experience. Living for the present is where your responsibility lies. Not dealing with negative sexual beliefs is a sure sign of a suppressed inner sexual passion wanting to be unleashed, but may be prevented because you might feel ashamed. Dealing with past influences on your sexual beliefs is a crucial first step because you need to become the sexual being God created you to be.

How do you overcome negative sexual beliefs?

You need to determine what the truth is about sex and Chapter 2 in *Between the Covers* is a good place to start. From there it should not be difficult to realise that God wants you to enjoy love making and have truly fulfilling sex with your spouse. He wants you to live out the biblical portrayal of sex and deliberately turn your back on all the negative sexual beliefs dragged from your past.

3.3 Pornography

Did you discover pornography at a very early age or maybe you just stumbled upon it one day and then became so fascinated with it that you wanted more and more? This is the danger of pornography; it is addictive.

The three main dangers of pornography in your marriage should be fully discussed before bringing it into your marriage. Pornography is firstly dangerous due to the images being imprinted in your mind. It is a way for sexual images of people other than your spouse to enter you mind and the risk is for those images to turn into fantasies. As seen in Chapter 2, the Bible clearly says in Matthew 5:28 that even lustfully thinking about someone other than your spouse is considered adultery. As a married Christian you should avoid pornography solely for this reason.

The byproduct is that these imprinted images turn into sexual fantasies while you are having sex with your spouse. It is unhealthy to have sex with your spouse, while fantasising about having sex with someone other than your partner. Even if the connotation of adultery is taken out of the equation, the issue still remains that your spouse deserves better from you. He or she deserves your full attention during sexual intercourse and thinking about anyone other than your spouse is taking away from what they deserve in your marriage. Pornography can become a dangerous threat to sexual fulfilment in your marriage.

The second danger of pornography in your marriage is its progression to sexual inability. You may think it will never happen to you, but eventually pornography leads to women being unable to reach orgasm and men experiencing impotence when trying to have sex with their spouses without using pornography as a sexual aid. In the beginning pornography might get you both in the mood and prepare you for sex, but using pornography over an extended period of time, you may eventually reach a point where you are unable to have sex without the use of pornography.

The third danger of pornography is its ever increasing craving for more; more and more pornography leads to physical actions like masturbation and eventually to sex with people other than your spouse. When you are focusing on pornography, you are subconsciously consenting to have sex with people other than your spouse and it may lead to you actually taking the step to make this a reality. Extramarital sex is the ultimate danger of pornography in your marriage.

You might not be using pornography at this point in your marriage or you may never have done so, but did you before you were married? If you did, it may still be affecting your marriage directly or indirectly. You may be measuring your spouse against the images you saw while you were using pornography and you may not even realise you are doing it. If you have ever used pornography, you should ensure you deal with it effectively so you do not carry the negative effects into your marriage.

How do you deal with it? Pornography directly affects your mind, so you need to deal with it on that level as the Bible recommends, saying you should 'be transformed (changed) by the [entire] renewal of your mind.'[45] This is done by confessing your sin, giving your mind to God and tenaciously avoiding any form of pornography, consequently keeping your mind pure.

3.4 Virginity

When did you lose your virginity? Were you a virgin on your wedding night? Did you lose your virginity to your spouse or did you lose it earlier in your life with someone else?

If you lost your virginity with someone other than your spouse, you will know how special the moment was because you gave away something very special to the other person. Why we are mentioning it here is because you probably still remember it. Losing your virginity is like your first kiss, you never forget it, but the dilemma comes in when you idealise your first sexual experience and begin to compare your spouse to it.

You might have been living a life filled with guilt because you lost your virginity before marriage with someone other than your spouse, but you cannot continue living like this because of the negative influence it will have on your spouse. Make peace with your past and put it behind you. This is a biblical principle and Paul said 'but one thing I do [it is my one aspiration]: forgetting what lies behind and straining forward to what lies ahead.'[46]

Yes, you lost your virginity with someone other than your spouse, but it is in the past. Do not lead the rest of your life based on past mistakes. Confess what needs confessing and deal with the guilt you might be experiencing, but then put it behind you and stop dwelling on the past. Focus your attention on your spouse and the present.

Every time you feel guilty about something from the past, it affects your marriage and your sex life, resulting in your inner sexual passion being hidden and you and your spouse losing out on true sexual fulfilment.

3.5 Premarital sex

When you lost your virginity outside of marriage, you might have made the decision to continue having sex because you had already lost your virginity. You probably thought that there was nothing left to protect and therefore continued having premarital sex; however, now you are married, you still feel guilty about all the previous sexual experiences you had or you compare your spouse to your previous sexual partners.

Premarital sex may also be a form of pornography in that you may be fantasising about previous sexual partners while having sex with your spouse. This is unfair to both you and your spouse and you should deal with it appropriately to ensure it is not negatively affecting your marriage and sex life.

But the biggest danger of premarital sex is the relationship aspects of your previous sexual partners. Does your spouse know them or know about them? Does your spouse ever have to mix with them because you still have contact with them and maybe still have them as your friends?

If so, you are being very selfish by making your spouse come into direct contact with your previous sexual partners. We advise that you break all ties with them in order to give your marriage and your spouse the necessary respect they deserve by not compelling your spouse to entertain your previous sexual partners. Never allow your premarital sexual experiences to influence your marital sex life in any way, not relationally and not by comparing your spouse to previous sexual partners; rather break all ties with them.

3.6 Sexual trauma

Sexual trauma includes rape, sexual molestation and sexual assault. You might have been the victim of such a heinous crime and act of violence against you. If you have, it might have been before your marriage or it might have been while you were already married. Sexual trauma is a major cause of your inner sexual passion being buried, but you do not want it hidden.

If you experienced sexual trauma in any form, it usually makes you feel dirty or sometimes guilty. It normally results in a fear of sex or promiscuity, but what it always leads to is the burial of your inner passion. It can also lead to you being promiscuous, having lots of sex and maybe with many partners, but this is not an unleashed inner passion because it is a result of tremendous hurt and pain. Your inner passion can only be truly unleashed when it is done with your spouse within the boundaries of your marriage as God intended it to be.

You might have been a virgin when you experienced sexual trauma and lost your virginity through a criminal act performed against you. This may still negatively affect your sex life as you see sex as a dirty and criminal act to be avoided. If you experienced sexual molestation as a child, you may have authority figure issues and may be sexually attracted to people younger than yourself because sex with an older person might remind you of the molestation. If you were sexually molested over an extended period of time, you are probably having spiritual and religious problems as you question God's love and will-ingness to protect you. You may also be hiding your inner passion if you see sex as dirty or, even worse, as a punishment from God.

It should come as no surprise that the negative effects of sexual trauma restrict your sexuality and withhold sexual fulfilment from you and your spouse because of this criminal action forced on you in your past.

Maybe you experienced sexual trauma after you got married. You might have been raped or sexually assaulted. Apart from the obvious and direct sexual consequences, it will also negatively affect your spouse. Your spouse might be feeling guilty for not preventing the sexual trauma, and feel personally responsible for the criminal offence against you. Unfortunately, there is no easy way to overcome sexual trauma.

If you have experienced sexual trauma in any form, seek professional help in effectively dealing with it, overcoming it and eliminating any remaining negative outcomes. Sexual trauma has a major negative influence on your marriage so you should make every effort to deal with it in the most appropriate manner.

As a Christian, make an appointment with an appropriately qualified pastoral therapist with more than enough experience in trauma counselling and especially sexual trauma. We suggest this type of therapist because of the spiritual dimension such a therapist will bring into the equation, thus effectively dealing with all affected aspects of your life.

Sexual trauma can be dealt with effectively, giving you a chance to go on with your life and find true sexual fulfilment in your marriage without allowing past trauma to direct your future.

3.7 Extramarital sex

You might have reached the point in your marriage where an extramarital affair seems very inviting. Perhaps the thought entered your mind because of pornography, due to unhappiness in your marriage or possibly because you wanted to experiment sexually, but your spouse's inner sexual passion has been hidden away so deeply that you thought extramarital sex was the only option.

If you as a married person have sex with someone other than your spouse, you must be aware of the dangers and especially of the resulting consequences of such an action. You will know how it feels to be classified as an adulterer even though no one else may be aware of it, but your guilty conscience has classified you as such. You will probably be aware of the guilt accompanying an extramarital affair, the fear of the affair becoming public knowledge as well as the shock, shame and moral breakdown you will experience as a result of the affair.

Extramarital sex directly affects your spouse and although your spouse may not be aware of what you are doing or have done, the consequences spill over into your marriage life and wedding bed. Your sex patterns change and your spouse does not know why.

Having had sex with someone other than your spouse also causes a connection to form between you and this third party in your marriage. You should take full responsibility for what you have done and make every possible effort to repair the damage. Confess the sin of adultery, break all ties with the person you had the affair with and cleanse your mind and life of all unrighteousness.

Most people who fall for the temptation of extramarital sex need help to effectively overcome it and the effects thereof. It is also very important to find out exactly what the reasons were for you becoming involved in an extramarital affair and to efficiently deal with these causes in order to prevent it from happening again. The next step will be to face up to the consequences, put the whole matter behind you and to continue with your life by making the decision to live a life worthy, holy and according to biblical principles instead of falling for sin and temptation.

3.8 Divorce

If you committed adultery and it eventually led to you being divorced, remember that your spouse had a valid and biblical reason for divorcing you, since Jesus said that adultery, unfaithfulness and sexual immorality are valid reasons for divorce.[47]

It should be said that although adultery is a valid reason for divorce, your spouse may decide to forgive you and give you a second chance, but this must be your spouse's decision to make.

Perhaps you and your spouse divorced for a reason totally different to adultery and sexual immorality. Divorce was never God's plan for your life, but because of his tremendous love for you, He is able to forgive you for the divorce; the sacrifice Jesus made for you is big enough to even forgive divorce. What should be done from your side is to confess your sin and the divorce or the reasons for the divorce. Then you should treat your ex-spouse with respect, even if it is difficult.

If you then commit yourself to a new spouse, break all emotional ties with your ex-spouse. You may not be able to break all ties with your ex-spouse because you've had children together, but you should break emotional ties so you will not have a clash of emotions.

Reassure your new spouse in word and in deed of your total commitment, regardless of having an ex-spouse. Never compare your spouse to your ex-spouse in any way, especially not when it comes to sex; rather just enjoy time with your new spouse and put everything into the relationship to make it work.

3.9 Summary

You are a sexual being and you have an inner sexual passion wanting to come out and play within your marriage. Your inner passion wants to be unleashed to experiment sexually and if done so in the correct manner, your spouse will be more than willing to experiment with you.

Your past has a definite influence on your sexual beliefs, attitudes and behaviours. What you believe from the past and what you have experienced in the past directly influences how you see sex at this point in your life.

If you are aware of how your past is manipulating your present regarding your sexuality, you will be in a much better position to compensate and to make an effort to deal with it. Your inner passion is hiding inside waiting for you to unleash it. If you effectively overcome all the objections, inhibitions and fears you have about sex based on what you have believed and experienced in your past, you will be able to unleash your inner passion in such a way as to encourage your spouse to do exactly the same.

Unleashing your inner sexual passion is necessary for you to find true sexual fulfilment in your marriage and to offer the same to your spouse.

CHAPTER 4

Sexual communication

Communication is the catalyst needed to unleash your inner passion and bring about positive change in your marriage. Doing this successfully begins with the ability to communicate effectively with your spouse about your sexual needs, wants, desires and turn-ons.

The perception that we are born with the ability to communicate efficiently is a myth and the reality is that everyone can be an excellent communicator. Communication skills can be learnt.

Without the ability to communicate well, people find it harder to succeed in life and in their careers. The same is true about marriage; good communication skills are needed to make a marriage work and to change your stale sexual relationship into the fulfilling one it was originally meant to be.

Communication is all about the ability to tell someone else exactly how you feel and what you want without coming across as pushy, while in return having the ability to really listen to what the other person is saying.

Good communication therefore begins with good listening skills and the ability to truly hear what your spouse is saying to you through words, behaviour, attitude and body language. To be able to really hear what your spouse is saying, you will have to learn how to hear what is being said between the lines; not listening to the words alone, but also to what is actually behind the words. Understanding why your spouse is saying something and the way your spouse is saying it is of great importance. To take it yet another step further, good listening skills also include the ability to hear what your spouse is not saying as well.

Body language is an excellent indicator of what is going on in your spouse's mind and effective listening skills will immediately help you to pick up on any discrepancies between your spouse's words and body language. The way a person acts says much more than the actual words, and if the words and body language do not correspond, the body language overrides the words. Being able to listen effectively will enable you to become aware of such inconsistencies and make it possible for you to ask the right questions and take the correct action.

Communication also refers to the ability to put your thoughts, needs, wants and desires into words in such a way as to ensure your spouse understands without doubt what you want and need. This is of the utmost importance in the process of unleashing your inner passion because your spouse is not a mind reader; to expect your spouse to know what you want and enjoy during sexual intercourse without actually sharing it is an unrealistic expectation.

Never expect your spouse to know what is going on in your mind, but rather make the effort to clearly talk about the matter at hand to ensure total understanding between the two of you. Silent treatment and trying to guess what your spouse wants and needs have never been an effective way to approach a marriage and your sexuality. Open communication is necessary between you and your spouse to ensure that both your inner passions are unleashed, resulting in marital sexual fulfilment.

4.1 Open communication

Open communication is the way in which you communicate with your spouse. This method does not allow misunderstandings, which may result in unnecessary resentment to creep in.

Communicating clearly about what you expect from your spouse is crucial if you desire a marriage and sexual relationship that both of you will fully enjoy. Your spouse does not have the ability to read your mind, so it is your responsibility to point out to your spouse exactly what your expectations are regarding your marriage, relationship and sex life.

Do you want your inner passion unleashed? Do you want to enjoy sex and experience real sexual fulfilment and orgasms of pleasure? Do you want your spouse to be able to take you into the starry heights of true sexual fulfilment and pleasure most of the time?

Then you will have to communicate openly with your spouse!

Being honest about sex, sexuality and your genitals may be a really scary thought and totally outside your comfort zone, but it is one of those vital things that must be done if you want to experience change and the resulting benefits.

If you are uncomfortable about communicating openly about your body and sexuality to your spouse, it is probably due to the way you grew up or due to being shy. Try to overcome these feelings and face up to your concerns if you truly want to experience the benefits of a sexually fulfilling marriage.

Hesitance in communicating openly about your sexuality and what you really want in the bedroom may cause frustration to build up and your unsatisfied sexual life to continue. It is possible to stop and break this cycle of unfulfilled sexuality, but the only way to do so is for you to talk to your spouse about it and then to put into practice some new ways and methods of approaching sexual intercourse.

If you do not tell your spouse you are unhappy and unfulfilled sexually, your spouse might not even realise it and think everything is perfect. Communication is needed to share your frustration with your spouse; not in a negative and degrading way, but rather by asking your spouse to help you become sexually fulfilled. Never make your spouse feel inadequate when it comes to sex, because it may only lead to feelings of rejection and inadequacy. Never make your spouse feel incompetent, especially when it comes to sexual intercourse, because it will lead to unnecessary hurt, pain and resentment towards you.

Open communication is the ability to share with your spouse exactly what is on your mind and in your heart regarding your sexuality, but without making your spouse feel incompetent and rejected. If you can develop this skill, you will be able to effectively communicate to your spouse what you need and want while at the same time releasing your inner passion and ensuring true sexual fulfilment in your marriage. Open communication is the heartbeat of a healthy marriage and sexual life.

4.2 Communicate about birth control

Every couple should talk about birth control, but this should be done before the wedding day. However, you may be married already and this topic has never been discussed; if this is the case, discuss this important subject without delay.

Why is it important to talk to your spouse about birth control?

The obvious answer is that when you are not in agreement about birth control and who is going to take responsibility for it, it may lead to pregnancy before you are ready for children. If you already have a child or children and one of them was unplanned, just realise that the child is a gift from God and although the little one arrived ahead of your planned time, he or she is still a blessing from God.

Birth control is the responsibility of both the husband and wife, but depending on the method decided on, one of the spouses will carry more responsibility. For example, if the decision has been made to use the birth control pill, making the decision is the responsibility of both the husband and the wife, but actually taking the pill, putting it in her mouth and swallowing it is the responsibility of the wife. The responsibility of the husband at this stage is to make sure his wife has actually taken the pill and keep her aware of products that might be affecting the effectiveness of the pill. This should be discussed with your family planning doctor, nurse or pharmacist, but it is usually things like antibiotics, certain painkillers and even not taking the pill at the same time every day.

There are many methods of birth control, ranging from condoms and diaphragms to implanted devices inside the wife, the not-so-effective method of coitus interruptus where the penis is withdrawn from the vagina just before ejaculation, all the way to more extreme measures like vasectomy or a hysterectomy.

Birth control should be discussed because the method used might affect the couple or one of the spouses. If you decide on the injection method, where an injection is given every few months, the wife should be aware that she will stop menstruating while she is on this birth control method and clearly understand how long it will take after she stops using it before she will be able to become pregnant. When using the birth control pill, the wife may have increased mood swings during certain times of her monthly cycle, which may possibly be more severe than they were before taking the pill.

It should be discussed and agreed upon by all couples, especially Christian couples, but as the authors we want to urge all couples, regardless of religion, not to make use of the morning-after pill. This is a method of birth control where a pill is taken the morning after sexual intercourse. The reason we do not recommended it is because this method does not prevent pregnancy, but rather aborts an already formed zygote after conception has taken place. We suggest that you use any form of birth control you and your spouse agree upon as long as it prevents conception rather than getting rid of an already conceived zygote!

Communication about birth control should also include a discussion about what will happen after you have all the children you want. Will you continue with the birth control method you used before you became pregnant or will you consider a permanent method like a vasectomy for the husband or a hysterectomy for the wife? This is a discussion not to be taken lightly and agreeing upon the way forward is of the utmost importance. It is a decision you will have to make as a couple, you should weigh up whether taking out the wife's organs during a hysterectomy is really the way you want to go or whether the husband should get a vasectomy instead. A vasectomy is not as severe and normal sexual function resumes more quickly.

4.3 Communicate about family planning

Family planning is the next topic you and your spouse should discuss, preferably before marriage. What a shock it will be if you want five children and your spouse does not want children at all, but because you never discussed it before your wedding day, you only found out after you had already committed to each other.

When talking about whether you want children or not, always justify your opinions with good reasons. Never just tell your spouse, for example, that you want two children and no more or no less, without giving a reason. True communication is being able and willing not only to share and converse about what you actually say, but also to consider the reasons behind your preferences.

At this point compromise is something both you and your spouse might want to consider. If the two of you cannot agree upon the number of children to have, negotiate till you reach an agreement or you will experience an unhappy marriage, resulting in children being raised in an unhappy home due to your inability or unwillingness to compromise.

The second aspect of communication about family planning is the conversation regarding the gender of your children. You are unable to determine the gender of the children God will give you, but you need to make a decision about how you will deal with this. If you, for example, only want two children, a boy and a girl, and God blesses you with two girls, how will you deal with it? Will you override your decision to only have two children and plan a third one, or will you be satisfied with your two girls and forget about the boy? This is an important discussion to have with your spouse.

4.4 Communicate about privacy during sex

Privacy is crucial during sex. You do not want to have sex fearing that someone will walk in while you are busy. This is especially important for couples with children. Having a child walk in while you are having sex is not only uncomfortable for you and your spouse but also uncomfortable for your child.

Privacy during sex is important, so you need to communicate about this, how you will deal with it and how you will ensure your privacy.

If you do have sex somewhere that is not private and someone may walk in on you at any time, you will have to live with the consequences! It is therefore suggested that you always have sex in private where you are sure of not being disturbed.

Does this mean you should not have sex with your spouse in public places? Well, this is exactly the type of communication you should have with your spouse. No one can make that decision for you, but you cannot make well informed decisions without the means of effective communication.

Another matter to discuss regarding privacy during sex is how private sex should be between you and your spouse. In other words, will you leave the light on during sex so your spouse can look at your body or will you want to switch the light off because you are shy about your body? This is a matter to discuss with your spouse and if either of you always want the light off, continue the conversation to discover why this is so and how it can be overcome, because your spouse may sometimes need and want to see you naked during sex.

4.5 Communicate about your sexual preferences and dislikes

If you do not tell your spouse what you like, dislike and prefer sexually it will be impossible for your spouse to know. Take responsibility for what you want and do not want and tell your spouse. If you are newlyweds, this might take time to determine, but communicate openly and honestly about what you dislike from the beginning to make it clear to your spouse.

Experimenting with different sexual positions should be preceded by open communication between you and your spouse. Discuss what positions to try out and what you think of them afterwards. If you do not like a certain position but do not tell your spouse, your spouse may want to continue using that specific position and it may lead to resentment from your side. To prevent this, rather tell your spouse exactly how you feel about it. Do not only tell your spouse yes or no about a sexual position, always give a reason or explanation for your answer.

If you do not like a position but your spouse does, how should this be handled? Communication may lead to a solution or agreement where you perhaps agree to be unselfish and have sex in the specific position just because your spouse enjoys it, but within limits. You may agree to use the position, but only once a month or every tenth time you have sex or whatever the two of you decide upon. You want your inner passion unleashed, but at the same time you want your spouse's inner passion unleashed as well. Being unselfish and sometimes (not every time, but sometimes) trying out new things like new sexual positions you might not particularly enjoy is a sign of a mature person and a mature marriage, where you provide a platform for your spouse to live out his or her sexual likes and desires. Your spouse should do exactly the same for you.

Open communication about sexual preferences should also include discussions about foreplay, sex during menstruation and these types of subjects. Never communicating about these things will either lead to you wondering how they could be or to resentment towards your spouse for requesting or expecting them from you.

Communication is crucial for you and your spouse to be on the same page when it comes to sexuality and your likes, dislikes and preferences.

4.6 Communication during sex

Do you like talking during sexual intercourse or do you want your spouse to talk to you during sex or foreplay?

Without discussing this with your spouse, neither of you will know what the other prefers and when there is a lack of communication regarding this, you may experience frustration until you take responsibility and start talking to your spouse.

Communication during foreplay can sometimes become part of the foreplay, obviously depending on what you talk about. Communication after sexual intercourse during the 'cooling down' period can be very intimate and may sometimes be a good time to really share your inner desires, hurts, fear or doubts with your spouse. Communication during sexual intercourse and while you are busy with the sexual act may be very erotic; whether you say actual words or just make noises and sounds will totally depend on you as a couple.

Discussing communication during sex is necessary to let you and your spouse's inner passions come out of the hidden depths of your desires and actually become a reality in your life and marriage.

4.7 Communicate about sexual quantity

How many times per week or per month are you going to have sex?

This is the question on the minds of numerous married couples. They all wonder what the normal quantity of sex is. Many of them may be thinking they are having far too little sex while their spouses may think they are having far too much sex.

On average, married couples have sex about three times per week, but every couple is different. Some married couples may have higher sex drives and probably have sex on a daily basis while others may have lower sex drives and only have sex once a week.

So for this reason you should communicate with your spouse about sexual quantity in your marriage and what is normal for you as a couple. Never compare yourself with other married couples or with anyone else; every couple is unique and you should discuss what the normal quantity of sex is for you as a couple.

What you should also communicate about is what happens when you have a different sex drive to your spouse. What will you do when you have a low sex drive and your spouse has a high sex drive? Or vice versa? Discuss this with your spouse and communicate until you reach an agreement about how this will be handled.

You may make the decision to always have sex when the other one wants it or you may decide to rather convert to oral sex during these times to provide relief to the one in need of sex. As a couple you have the option of bringing masturbation or the use of sexual toys into this equation.

Whatever you decide as a couple, it can only be decided upon after you talk about it. Without communication it will be impossible for you to make a decision about sexual quantity.

What should never be done, however, is to reject your spouse. When you do not have a need for sex, but your spouse does, you should never reject your spouse and just ignore him or her, because then you open the door for the enemy to move into your marriage and start tempting your spouse to look elsewhere. This could be true for you too if you are the one with the higher sex drive and your spouse does not want sex. This is not an excuse for either of you to have an extramarital affair, but it increases the possibility of such behaviour.

Opening the door to the enemy of sexual temptation should never be allowed by any married couple. Sexual quantity is a very real threat for your marriage and definitely one of the most evident ways of giving the enemy a permanent room in your marriage.

Having sex should always be fun and if your inner passion is unleashed, you will truly enjoy it and at the same time, be willing to have sex even when you are not in the mood, just to spoil your spouse. This is what true marriage is all about; unselfishness and the ability to make your spouse happy and fulfil their very basic needs and wants.

Communication about sexual quantity is a very real discussion every married couple should have as soon as possible after the wedding or even before the wedding day. Once each spouse knows what their own needs and wants are for sexual quantity, as well as the needs and wants of their spouse, they can accommodate these differences in the marriage. Newlyweds might not know yet what the optimal quantity for them will be, but communication about this even before marriage is important in order for both to know what the general idea or expectation is about sexual quantity.

4.8 Communicate about sexual quality

After deciding on the sexual quantity for your marriage and for you as a married couple, discuss what you see as quality sex. Sex is not only about quantity, but definitely about quality as well. What do you see as good sex and what does your spouse see as good sex?

You should realise the quality of sex may also have an influence on the sexual quantity. If your spouse wants sex more than you do, it may not be because your spouse has a higher sex drive than you do, but because the sex your spouse is receiving from you is of such a low quality that your spouse is trying to make up for that by sexual quantity. When you therefore begin to have quality sex, your spouse's sex drive might even decrease slightly, thus accommodating both of you in quality and quantity.

The only way to determine what your spouse views as quality sex is through communication.

Unleashing your inner passion will ensure you are adventurous in the bedroom and are willing to experiment sexually with various positions and different methods. This will bring excitement into your sex life, leading to both you and your spouse experiencing true sexual fulfilment.

Quality sex begins with communication, with both you and your spouse talking to each other and discussing what you want and need sexually, and how you will be able to make it a reality in your marriage.

4.9 Communicate about absence

Modern society is a very fast-paced environment and often leads to a spouse being absent, either due to travelling for work or working away from home for weeks on end. How is this absence of a spouse handled? It is a very important topic of discussion to be dealt with if you want your marriage to survive these absences.

Modern society is not only fast paced, but also technologically evolved and there are numerous ways to keep your inner passion unleashed while still staying faithful to your spouse and not allowing the enemy of temptation to enter your mind, your marriage or your sexual life.

Communication about the absence of a spouse should include discussion about what you and your spouse's sexual needs will be during the period of absence or distance between you, and how you will deal with them in the most effective way and in a way approved by both of you.

You can discuss the possibility of phone sex where the telephone is used between the two of you to talk about sex with each other, or you may decide to abstain from sex for the full duration of the absence of the spouse.

Another option is cyber sex between you and your spouse where modern technology like a computer, webcam and microphone or even a webcam enabled cellular phone is used to have online sex. This can be described as sex over a distance where you look at each other on the webcam while talking to each other and possibly even go so far as to get undressed and mutually masturbate. The only difference is it is done between you and your spouse while you are away from each other instead of being in the same room or in the same bed. How you handle absence can only be dealt with through open and honest communication, and you should both be comfortable with whatever you decide, whether engaging in phone sex, cyber sex or abstinence for the limited period.

4.10 Summary

Communication is the heartbeat of every marriage and every married couple's fulfilled sexual desires.

Married couples should spend time learning communication and listening skills and then put them into practice by setting time apart to communicate with their spouses. Without open and honest discussions taking place between you, there is no way for your spouse to understand you or you to fully understand your spouse.

Both you and your spouse have certain sexual preferences, desires, wants, likes and dislikes. The only way to understand what your spouse wants is to effectively listen to what he or she says and to clearly communicate to your partner what you want.

Communication is much more than just listening to your spouse's words and then for your spouse to listen to your words. It is also about clearly talking and listening while your attitude, body language and words all agree with each other, noting any discrepancies between them.

Unleashing your inner passion is possible and attainable when you learn the art of communication and actually put it into practice in your daily life and in your interaction with your spouse.

CHAPTER 5

Unique sexuality

5.1 Personality and temperament and how it influences your sex life

Every human being is a unique creation and each individual has their own temperament, personality, likes and dislikes, developmental phases and so on.

God used the same template when He created us but He made us so that we function very differently. Every person is special but you were not created to be a unique superior being; you were created to serve God through being individually unique. So do not compare yourself to other people or try to become like other people because it is not what God created you to be. Rather develop into the unique person God created you to be and continue to serve Him. Begin doing this by focusing on the good and the positive in your own life.

Every woman has breasts, a clitoris, vagina and anus. Every man has nipples, a penis and an anus. How each individual looks and performs is different, however. Some people might have a different amount and colour of pubic hair, some a clitoris more covered by a hood than others, penis sizes vary, pelvis sizes vary, and different people have different sensual spots and react differently to various sexual interactions. For instance, you might stroke satin over your spouse's skin, but you might not like the feeling of satin material against your own skin. These differences make us uniquely beautiful yet very normal.

A frequently asked question is about the sexual bodily fluids from the vagina or the penis. This is very unique to every person. A woman's vagina may not be able to produce the amount of fluids necessary to perform comfortable sexual intercourse, so you will have to accommodate the situation by making use of water-based lubricant gel. On the other hand, her vagina may produce so much fluid that you might feel a little lost. All of this is very normal and you should be able to find a way to accommodate both of you without a serious problem.

A man may sometimes ejaculate more fluids than at other times. This is normal, even though it is unique to him. The media is very outspoken about sexual intercourse but it tends to ignore the detail you need most: you are the way you should be. You are perfectly created by your Creator. Some products and services on the market are simply not needed as the adverts imply.

If you believe your penis is not big enough, work on your belief and technique, not the size of your penis. If you believe your breasts are not perfect, comfortableness is what you should be looking for. Before considering surgery, think it through carefully. Changes to the body bring adjustments to your lifestyle and may later cause you to live uncomfortably. The same is true when you do not live healthily. To get final clarity about surgery, prayer is the wise thing to do.

As a matter of interest, surgery is available for women struggling to reach clitoral orgasm. This is a medically performed surgery where the hood of the clitoris is split. But first consult with a medical professional and try out less invasive procedures and methods.

Pregnancy is a unique sexual situation and the most beautiful time in a couple's marriage. You may have sex during the full term of pregnancy unless you have your doctor's recommendation not to do so. Sexual positions need to be adjusted to make it as comfortable as possible. For instance, the missionary position will not be possible in later months. Sexual intercourse will not complicate the pregnancy or hurt the baby in any way. We suggest a few positions to accommodate your pregnancy. The love you show towards a pregnant wife is just as important as when she is not pregnant. As a matter of fact, loving interaction will allow for positive growth for the infant.

You will never reach the point of loving too much. You may love as much as you want to! Remember, there is a difference between spoiling someone and loving someone. Spoiling does not fill the empty spaces where love is needed.

There is a war going on in the spiritual realm and part of the fight is for your body. God created us in his perfect image, but the enemy wants to make you believe you are worthless and make you feel unhappy about yourself. The enemy hates it when you are happy with yourself and you are using your perfectly created body to serve God and love your spouse. The enemy wants you to worry about how much bodily fluids are produced, whether you are good enough in bed and whether you are made in proportion, and then he makes you insecure by letting you compare yourself to friends and movies or pictures. You need to come to terms with being unique and you should move forward by enjoying yourself with your spouse through the help of the Holy Spirit. Being created in God's image is a privilege.

The objective of living a godly lifestyle is more important than constantly focusing on the problematic areas needing attention. Change your personal lifestyle to accommodate God's abundance and then move forward and ask Him to supply you with what you need.

Love each other; husband, take the lead and love your wife. Tell your wife you love her; she wants to hear it. Hold her, touch her, put your arm around her, and hold her hand. Kiss her, hold her leg when she sits next to you, scratch her back, kiss her hello, kiss her goodbye and hug her regularly. Give her things to show her you love her; buy flowers, chocolates, teddy bears, hearts, balloons and whatever will show her you love her. Give her a massage, talk to her about herself, sing to her, write a poem, leave her to sleep late, give her a foot massage, take her with you, spend time with her, encourage her, approve of her, tell her you are proud of her and make her feel like the number one person in every situation. Introduce her to your colleagues and tell her how beautiful she is. Make her feel like the most precious person in your life.

When your sex life seems down and out, take a new approach towards it and believe it can be how you want it to be. Then approach making love with your spouse in the same manner you have imagined. Many things change and become better when we become enthusiastic about them and involve our spouse. When you want to make love, clearly indicate this to your spouse in a kind manner.

Most women are taught from childhood to respect a man's ego and never to tell him when she is unsatisfied or when she sees him making mistakes. This is why the truth will set you free. As an adult, it is easier to tell your husband how to satisfy your sexual needs and to find out how to satisfy his sexual needs. It is not perverse and it is not difficult after you know how. Even after your spouse knows exactly what you would like them to do, you need to practise it and this is where the fun part starts!

Try out our suggestions and you might be pleasantly surprised at the positive change in your sex life. If you do not find the passion returning to your marital sex life, something else might need work and can be rectified with prayer and counselling.

Mature, humble marriages allow for success and prosperity to be part of them. Use whatever potential your spouse has and develop it. When he or she wants to try something new, do not discourage them in case it might embarrass you; try to be open minded and trusting in the new venture.

You know your spouse's weaknesses better than anyone else. God entrusts you with such intimate information so that you can stand strong in the gap for your spouse without seeking approval for it or defeat your spouse with it. In the same way that God loves it when you are secretively good to someone without boasting, this is an opportunity to bring glory to his Name.

The way you are is the way you make love. When you look at a person and see their uniqueness, it will be exactly the way they make love in bed. So the way your life reflects who you are will also reflect the way you make love. Are you lazy by nature? Then you are probably lazy during sexual intimacy as well. This is often why great achievers are really popular with the opposite sex. The important point to realise is you are what you chose to become, so choose to be different, act differently and behave differently and soon your life and sex life will be different.

What is a mature marriage? It is a safe relationship with a forgiveness measure of 70 times seven, unlimited understanding, caring, compassion (a place to make mistakes and a place to grow), respect, privacy and passion towards each other for one reason only, because of your love for Jesus Christ.

Your friendship and your sex life with your spouse will both be unique. To compare it to someone else's sex life and their marriage would be tearing yours down. Explore and find the uniqueness of your own marriage and the uniqueness between you and your spouse. You will not be happier with someone else's marriage or sex life or even with their sex style.

When you enter into marriage, your objective is to serve our Saviour, Jesus Christ. Marriage and love are choices you make with both your mind and your heart, being well aware of what you are doing. If this is not the way your marriage is, let your marriage belong to God and work for Him. In this way the responsibility of keeping your spouse happy and satisfied does not seem overwhelming but possible, because now you can turn to God when your spouse needs something and ask his assistance.

Do not expect from God what you are not willing to give Him. In other words, do not ask God for a great sex life and then not be prepared for God to enter your mind and even be in your mind while making love. When you are led by the Holy Spirit you need only ask and his help will be available.

This is never so needed as when your spouse wants to experiment sexually with something and you do not. Sometimes you will have to do things you do not want to just to make your spouse happy, but this should always be done under the guidance of the Holy Spirit and not against the will of God.

Unique sexuality is even more; it is where a husband and wife do not discuss each other's weaknesses or private matters with strangers; only with the Holy Spirit. Do not share your sexual information with other couples or individuals in conversation since it causes complications you will find difficult to deal with later. Should you already have done so, ask your spouse's forgiveness and make the decision not to do it again. Difficult matters can be discussed with a physician, counsellor or a church leader, but preferably always with your spouse's knowledge and/or permission.

It is one thing to joke and you can sometimes even get a bit scruffy, but always have your spouse's best interest at heart and never make your spouse feel degraded, hurt or embarrassed.

Be careful not to act overly jealous towards your spouse, never allowing him or her freedom to enjoy life; rather purposely start right now and learn ways to have your spouse's positive loving attention. Believe in what you are capable of and the wonderful love God put in your life and reflect it into your relationship and sex life.

The enemy knows your bad personality traits, knows what makes you mad, sad or feel terrible. Do not feed yourself to the enemy. When you cannot get control of your anger or jealousy, tell God immediately. Pray in the spirit and get control of your emotions. Jealousy equals hurting your relationship.

Be kind to all people, but mostly be kind to your spouse. Practise this and make it part of your lifestyle. You are there to help build your spouse. What you say about your spouse and your marriage is the blessings or curses that will happen, should one or both of you believe it. What are you consciously or unconsciously telling other people about your marriage? What are you saying about your spouse without using words? Do you show you approve of them and love them? Do you show you are happy in your marriage? Are you proud to have such a wonderful spouse? Do you thank God every morning for the spouse whom you chose and with whom He entrusted you?

Uniqueness is built over time, making good memories, and things to remember and talk about later between you and your spouse. Building uniqueness takes regular practise and ideas, no matter how big or small they are.

It is really good to live a holy life, but do not have a holier-than-thou attitude in the bedroom. Playing, laughing and being silly together in the bedroom when the two of you are alone is not only necessary for a healthy marriage, but it serves as a building block for the future of the marriage. Laughing together is fun! You do not have to have sex; you can play together and let sex happen when it happens.

What kind of fun would you like to have with your spouse for you to keep in your memory bank? Initiate some play-time with your spouse and then see how you both begin to enjoy each other and spending more time with each other.

5.2 Cultural differences influence sexuality

Different cultures have different ways of doing things, like preparing food, dressing, marrying, training the children and communicating. When two people enter into a cross-cultural marriage, they not only have to adapt to each other's differences but also the differences in culture.

Each individual should be accommodated according to their physical build. Should a man have a large penis and be married to a wife with a small vagina, they should talk about the regularity of sexual intercourse.

Certain cultures practice female genital mutilation, a procedure of removing a little girl's clitoris at the age of five, supposedly to please her husband one day. In Western countries this is a criminal offence with jail time of up to 40 years.[48]

We may question what the reason is behind this practice and why it is done to young children. Is it a lack of trust; fear of humiliation due to premarital sex; perception of pleasure being sin; wrong spiritual beliefs of seeing sex only as a means of reproduction and not for sexual pleasure, or is it a cultural ritualistic activity performed without having a valid reason for actually doing it? When the reason is determined, it is not difficult to conclude where the practice originated and how to effectively resolve it, and in the process allow young girls to grow up to also experience sexual pleasure in their marriages.

Maybe you are the woman who has been disrespected in this way and now you are married but unable to experience any pleasure from sexual activity. You may be really frustrated and unaware of how to overcome the situation or how you will ever be able to experience sexual pleasure in your marriage.

A medical examination is a possible first step to see if there is physically anything to be done to help you experience sexual pleasure again. The second step will be to experiment with some alternative ways of having sex, finding pleasure in closeness, sensuality and the touch of your loving husband. The third step is, along with your husband, to experiment with your body to determine what sensitive areas cause you pleasure and then to especially focus on those areas during sexual activity. The fourth step is to forgive your perpetrators and put the past behind you by making the decision to live for the present and not stay locked up in the negative experiences of the past. The fifth and most important step is to allow God to touch you, renew your mind and with his help make a success of your marriage and your situation.

5.3 Difficult circumstances influencing your sex life

Despite all the circumstances that a marriage can endure, it is important to also remember each spouse's individual growth towards maturity.

When you enter into marriage, you accept your spouse the way he or she is. The most difficult thing you can do, is to try to change your spouse. You will only end up being disappointed and your spouse will feel like a miserable failure. Question your motives: what precisely do you expect from changing your spouse, because this is definitely a wanting from your side not your spouse's? If you tell your spouse the reason for your concerns, pray before taking a matter to him or her. God is in the business of changing people. He can do more for you and your spouse than you can.

Today's society offers many challenges to a marriage. You can change anything and everything but it is important and your responsibility to live with God in your life and to take care of yourself. Be awake and assertive, be patient as time allows the truth to emerge. Maturity heals difficulties in a marriage.

One of the purposes of marriage is for you to become sexually honest with yourself and with your spouse, so that you may be set free and enjoy it. It is a process to accomplish open and honest communication in marriage and especially your sex life, but when you achieve this you will become the best sexual partner ever. Remember to practise and practise!

Without warning a storm can arise in your lives and it has to be dealt with. By storm we refer to a difficult or unbearable situation so that the sex act is either heavily implicated or stopped.

So what kind of things can reduce your sex life? HIV/Aids, sexually transmitted diseases, accidents, loss of a job, being depressed, death of a child, being traumatised, difficult financial situations, debt, ill health, medical disorders, eating disorders, physical disabilities, bad timing, incredibly high expectations, poor personal hygiene, lack of intimacy and romance, fighting, contradictory beliefs, bad habits and addictions, fatigue, being overworked, different working hours, stress, poor self-esteem and influences of many other kinds.

To rid your sex life of these influences you need to clear your list of things to do and put your faith in God. Read the Bible with more quantity and quality, contemplating the Word of God for your daily life and after giving God first place in your life, give your spouse second place. When you, God and your spouse join forces, there is just no way for any bad circumstances to have any ground in your lives. It might take time identifying the exact characteristics of your problem: dedication, long suffering, patience, but with God there is a way to solve those problems. The bond between you, God and your spouse should carry priority over your sex life with your spouse, because God gave sex for enjoyment of each other, but only after enjoying his presence in your life.

Some men have high expectations about their sexual performance in the bedroom, but even if a man does not perform as he expected, it does not make him less of a man. A wife will not reject her husband or even love him less just because he was unable to perform sexually. This is when open communication and honesty is essential. The wife may tell her husband when she needs to engage sexually and give him some time to prepare for it and then she may make use of sex toys or intimate cuddling. Having problems in your sex life can be devastating, but it is always possible to overcome these obstacles with love, dedication, patience, creativity and honest communication.

If divorce has entered your mind, it is not the end of your marriage; it simply indicates a really big underlying marriage problem. It always feels like a way out, maybe even an answer in desperate circumstances and an excellent threatening tool.

Divorce is a very cruel measure where people end up getting hurt. Divorce is only meant to be a solution for people who need to get out of an adulterous marriage.

It was meant to be a protective tool which changed through time into a destructive and threatening tool. Never entertain the thought of divorce in your marriage and do not fear it either; when it arises from the heart of your spouse, deal with it by getting God involved. You need to remember that God is real and is with you always.[49] Ask God to help you rise above the situation and see the kingdom perspective of the problem. Address the problem with his help, not to go against your spouse but to help you both resolve the problem in reverence to God. Never go into a situation without God, no matter how ugly it gets!

It's sometimes difficult for a very private person to discuss sexual desires with a spouse. This is understandable and should be respected; however, every effort should be made to bring sexual intercourse to fulfilment for both spouses. Remember God gave both you and your spouse the promise of sexual enjoyment and fulfilment in marriage.

Fights are the most common denominator for crashing a well planned sexual evening. Does it matter if you are right or if you are wrong? Who will remember tomorrow or in a week's time or in a year's time? Just let it go and say you are sorry (you need to practise this to become really good at it). Remember that make-up sex is a great come-back from a bad experience!

Women have risen in communities and business. This has put a lot of pressure on them, especially in third world countries where men still expect to be served by their wives at their request. In first world countries where both husbands and wives work, both do household chores and both help in raising their children, seeing to their needs together. Both spouses contribute towards the expenses and both want to grow and do well in their future together. Should you be living in a third world country, it would be wise for you to try to entertain a first world standard. In this way both spouses have less stress and pressure and they are both free to love and respect each other as best they can. There are less expectations to be met and growth for both individuals in the marriage and business is the order of the day.

Abuse in any form is destructive. Whether you abuse to protect, to control, to save or for any other reason, there is never a good excuse for it. Abuse strangles love and it is sure to destroy sexual intimacy. If your spouse makes love to you after you have abused them, it will never be out of love, it will be out of fear. Relationships deteriorate after abuse and will keep on deteriorating until such time the couple call on God's help. After calling on God, the relationship will go through a process of healing which means it will need time to build up trust, respect, commitment and love. Love should be restored in your relationship through forgiveness, together with faith and hope through ongoing honest and kind actions.

It is hard to say you are sorry when you are not used to it; start practising it the next time the enemy tries to steal from your sex life. Remember, to be able to make a fight work, at least two people should be involved, so if one stops, the fight is dissolved. Diffuse the situation and discuss the real problem when you are both calm enough to think before you say something hurtful. Be the first to refuse to fight, and deal maturely with all issues by means of open and mature communication.

Negative thought patterns can impact your sex life tremendously. You may experience impotence or the inability to reach orgasm and then become so focused on the problem that you forget to enjoy the sexual experience itself. Do not allow fear or disappointment to rob you of intimacy with your spouse. Enjoy each other without any pressure; relax and do not fear. You may try again once you are completely relaxed and your mind is focused on your spouse instead of on the problem. Should you still encounter difficulty, do not give up, cuddle your spouse and end the experience pleasantly without blame. You need something to look forward to next time and not to be afraid. Should the problem persist, you might want to consult a medical physician.

Obesity may cause difficulty and limit sexual fulfilment due to certain positions being uncomfortable, depth of penetration being inadequate and sometimes a lack of energy making sexual intercourse difficult. If you or your spouse struggle with obesity it is recommended that you do whatever is necessary to lose the excess weight in order to improve your health and sex life.

Friends and family may cause unnecessary strain on a marriage, especially if they are living in the same house. Remember, your spouse is your first priority after God and therefore you should never allow friends and family to affect your marriage relationship negatively. The Bible is very clear about people leaving their families and clinging to each other when they get married.[50] It is very important to always make your spouse feel secure by never allowing friends or family to interfere in the marriage. Always commit to your spouse, because when everyone goes home you do not want to sleep alone; you want to sleep next to your spouse.

In life you can be sure of only one thing and that is God. Friends, family and everything else will move on and eventually pass on; it is how life goes. Your spouse has been given to you by God to have, to hold and to enjoy for life. Your spouse will most probably be by your side for longer than anyone else. A positive investment into your attitude towards your spouse and into your relationship will build good, strong memories.

No friendship or relationship is worth your time or effort if it does not respect your marriage or spouse. Your priority is with your marriage as you made a commitment before the Lord regarding your spouse. It is your responsibility to keep your marriage stronger than any other friendship and you might be surprised how intimacy between you and your spouse blooms.

Letting go of manipulating friendships and bad habits will help your marriage to become strong.

5.4 Distance and its influence on your sex life

Distance in marriage has become a very familiar phenomenon. In modern-day society husbands and wives often live apart for various reasons and circumstances. Some of these marriages withstand the distance and still survive.

These spouses develop their own individuality more than they would develop as one, but it is not recommended, as it is not a building stone for the marriage. Even though these partners find it possible to live this way, they have to work harder to keep their marriages strong. What becomes a real challenge in a marriage where spouses are separated by distance is keeping the passion and desire alive, and still being faithful to each other.

You can enjoy foreplay by making use of cell phones and Internet calls during the week, while waiting for the weekend when you can be together at home.

If you tend to be suspicious about the faithfulness of your spouse, consciously make the decision to trust him or her unless you have proof of your partner being unfaithful. Do not allow any negative thoughts about your spouse into your mind during the time apart and rather focus on your spouse's good qualities. Negative thoughts will have a negative effect on your system and, over a long period of time, may result in emotional and physical illness.

Make the conscious decision to be happy with your spouse and to not want anyone else for any reason. Stop worrying about what your spouse may or may not be up to and live your life and marriage dedicated to the Lord, because if your spouse has something to hide it will eventually be revealed; do not waste your time worrying about it.

5.5 Summary

In this day and age your marriage has to withstand many circumstances and influences. But your marriage is uniquely special before the Lord and you need to focus on your own circumstances within your marriage and lay them before the Lord in prayer. You need to know that you and your spouse are following the Bible, which is the Word of God, and that you are submitting to the Holy Spirit.

Only take advice about your marriage from a person who knows God, who stands in a successful marriage and is the same gender as yourself, a person who steadfastly believes in God and believes positively in your marriage. Bless your marriage regularly and pray for your marriage.

Use ideas from the Bible to pray into your marriage. Christians call it praying Scripture. The Bible is packed with great ideas to pray for praying with a purpose. Some examples of such Scriptures are found in: Proverbs 5:18; 12:4; 18:22; 19:14; 31:11; Ecclesiastes 9:9 and Ephesians 5:33.

Being married to a spouse who does not believe in Jesus can possibly complicate your sex life. Focus on building your faith to give God glory as a first priority and then please your spouse in the flesh as a second priority. The spirit seeks to please God and the flesh seeks to please itself.

How do you know if you are able to make your spouse believe in

God? You do not know, so you can only pray and believe. God saves people, you do not. Your spouse chooses for him- or herself to follow God. God blesses whom He chooses, when and how He chooses. When God blesses you, enjoy it! Believe in Him, love Him, and enjoy his blessing when it comes your way.

CHAPTER 6

Gender

6.1 Husbands and sex

Men and women view sex very differently. Women see sex as an emotional experience of closeness with their husbands and as the ultimate expression of their love. Men, on the other hand, see sex as a physical experience of tension relief and pleasure.

Husbands approach sex accordingly; as a physical act of pleasure and as men they are always ready for sex and constantly thinking about sex. Wives, however, need some time to get ready for sex and therefore husbands should spend time throughout the day loving their wives, touching them and flirting with them. Women need to know their husbands love them and without the assurance of their love and commitment, sex will never be a completely fulfill sexual desires.

Why is this even mentioned? Husbands should be aware of the difference between their own approach to sex and that of their wives. This knowledge of how husbands and wives differ from each other provides valuable guidelines on how to approach your spouse and ensure sexual fulfilment.

Unleashing your inner passion is different for husbands than for wives. Husbands generally want more sexual *quantity* while wives require more sexual *quality*. Ensuring the unleashing of both the husband and wife's inner passion is a process of collaboration to ensure sexual quality as well as quantity. Together husbands and wives are able to overcome their different points of view regarding sex and work together to make it the ultimate experience of pleasure, intimacy and sexual fulfilment.

Wives should become aware of their husbands' constant need for sexual intercourse and discontinue using sex as a weapon to manipulate. Women should realise their husbands need sex and when they are sexually fulfilled, there will be no need for them to ever look around for other women. Husbands should realise this as well, because if they keep their wives sexually fulfilled there will be no need for them to ever look at other men. This does not place the responsibility for sexual purity on your spouse, but it does make your spouse aware of your own sexual needs and desires.

Never use your gender as an excuse or reason to abuse your own sexuality. It is your responsibility to live a life of sexual purity and dedication to your spouse without allowing your eyes, minds and bodies to wander. Live sexually pure lives and you will experience true happiness and fulfilment with your spouse.

Become aware of your gender and how it influences your general behaviour as well as your sexual behaviour. Compare your own behaviour and sexual needs to your spouse's to give you a clear understanding of how to act towards your spouse to ensure sexual fulfilment in your own life as well as in the life of your partner.

Husbands, take the responsibility to become sexually sensitive to your wives' needs and fulfil them. Wives, use your femininity to live out your sexuality while meeting your husbands' needs. In this way you will focus on unleashing the inner passion in your spouse without selfishness.

Changes in today's society have resulted in husbands facing numerous challenges, making it difficult but not impossible to truly be the ideal husband. The ideal husband is the one fulfilling his wife's specific needs. Remember the awesomeness of God who knows the needs and accomplishments of every individual. He knows the thoughts of your heart, the very pulsing of your desires. No matter how low you think you might be on the list of importance, you are number one on God's list because you were made in his Image. Do not allow circumstances to steal your joy or enjoyment of life, and that includes your sex life.

Enjoy life, not merely drawing from happiness, because happiness has a beginning and an end, the same as sadness. Engage in joy, because joy is a spiritual fruit not influenced by circumstances, but a deep-seated knowing. If you feel a bit down, consciously make the decision to rekindle your joy.

There is a huge difference between childishness and being childlike. Childishness is being foolishly immature. Being childlike is being youthful and encouragingly energetic, playful and kind. Your childlikeness is attractive to your spouse; do not bury it under the toolbox in the garage, but rather get it out, dust it off, polish it and use it. It will most probably help your wife to find her childlike or playful side and unleash it as well.

The greatest memories a woman will always speak about are those actions she did not plan. Actions like when her husband was playful and did something unexpected for her or with her; where he suddenly started enjoying her and enjoying life. You need one joyful thought to trample all your troublesome thoughts. No amount of trouble can ever kill joy; the only thing killing joy is the decision only you can make. Not even crooked teeth can spoil a great smile!

There is also a big difference between being insecure and being humble. Insecurity answers to people and has unreliable results. Humility answers to God and it has great results. The way to get rid of insecurities is, under the Holy Spirit's guidance, to become knowledgeable about the subject or object causing you to feel insecure and then to overcome it and to move on. When the enemy reminds you about it, remind him you have already conquered it through Jesus Christ.

Never compare yourself with other spouses or married couples. You are unique, God created you like that, and you are special to your husband or wife. Comparing yourself to others will only lower your self-image. What you should do instead is to focus on your good qualities and attributes, use them and develop them. A man developing his marriage and his love for his wife is like the sun shining on a mirror. The mirror portrays the role of the wife and she reflects what the husband sows into her and the marriage.

A good quality to develop, promising to make your life more enjoyable, is to love your wife unconditionally. Love her and make her feel loved. Love her and praise her for loving the Lord. Love her respectfully above all other women, including your mother and her mother. Love her in private and love her in public by respecting her and treating her accordingly in the way you talk to her and about her. Love her when she makes a mistake and love her even more when she is so unlovable. Why? God enables you to love her. Tell her you love her when she is mean and unkind, when she does not deserve it, and say it like you mean it. Love her when she is busy, bored, annoying, careless, wonderful, respecting, weak and strong. Love her even when she is not with you and you speak on the phone, love her in your thoughts. Teach the kids to love and respect her and when they forget remind them, again and again. Love the Lord and show her you love the Lord by praying with her and reading the Bible with her. Show your wife how and where you can see God loves her.

There is a well-known axiom stating 'a lion is a lion even when he sleeps'. It is so true. You are the husband in your marriage and no one can take that away from you. Problems and disappointments cannot take it from you. Circumstances cannot take it from you. Even when you fall down, are weak, sick or disabled, you are still the husband and you should live your life accordingly.

You may have been hurt by life and in your relationships and you did not deserve it, but do not allow past hurt to affect your life and future. Healing is possible and it usually starts with forgiveness. Forgive whoever needs to be forgiven and do not allow unforgiveness and past hurt to influence you negatively.

Many things may influence you; your work, circumstances in life, financial matters and many more, but never allow circumstances to dictate your sexual life and the way you behave towards your wife.

Husbands, let us talk briefly about a matter few people want to address. What happens when you are the one with the lower sex drive and your wife has a need for more sex than you do? How do you deal with your wife's greater need for sex when you physically cannot keep up? Does it make you feel inadequate in the bedroom? Does it make you feel incompetent in the sex department? Do you fear you will not be able to satisfy your wife sexually, resulting in her looking for sexual fulfilment elsewhere?

These are all very relevant questions and questions husbands would rather ignore than face head on.

Husband, you should realise you are the man your wife chose. You are exactly what she wants and if her sex drive is higher than yours, she would rather you dealt with it as a couple than find someone else to fulfil her needs. So, lift up your head, look these questions in the eye and acknowledge where you are right now in your marriage. If you cannot physically keep up with your wife's sexual desires, communicate openly about it with her and generate a plan of action as a couple. You might want to consider a sex toy or you might want to think outside the box by realising that you do not have to have full intercourse in order to fulfil your wife's needs. There are many other ways to do it as well, but what will work for you as a couple? Openly discuss this with your wife.

What is hidden is always a problem, but as soon as you reveal it to your spouse, the two of you will be able to deal with it appropriately and all of a sudden it will not be an issue anymore.

Husbands, you may have real fears and concerns about sex but usually hide them under macho bravado. You are not the only man having those concerns, many others do as well and instead of living a life concerned about these things, rather reveal them to your spouse so the two of you may handle them appropriately in a way that unleashes the inner passion in both of you.

6.2 Wives and sex

There has been a definite change in the last couple of decades in the realm of women. Up until fairly recently, women had no rights at all.

They did not have the privilege of having an identity or expressing an emotion or opinion. Women could not vote or even have a baby without a man's consent. They could not open bank accounts, own property or get driver's licences, except when it served the husband's needs. Today things are different and women are educated, successful, independent and free. The majority of women have made this their lifestyle.

Women have earned the responsibility of keeping their femininity intact and have the choice to humbly submit to their husbands, respecting them for their physical and spiritual protection. Women assist their husbands by being fierce spiritual warriors for the home and when women fall, they get up and press forward. Today's women are truly women of valour.

We believe the battle in the bedroom has been won as well. Years ago the majority of women did not have a choice whether they wanted to have sex or not. Now it has changed. Women rejoice in being Kingdom divas. They love passionately, flirting with their husbands with text messages, gifts, surprises, sexy underwear, teasing smiles, homemade food in candlelight and even as they get older they hold hands and stay true to their one and only.

In first world countries, women have learnt to share responsibilities with their husbands and children. This serves them well, because they are not stressed to a point of avoiding sexual contact. When they relax, they are able to enjoy marriage to the full by having enough energy for sexual intercourse.

It is important to know that God made the sexual act for mature adults to enjoy spontaneously. An immature person may miss the ingredients necessary for sexual fulfilment. When you are performing as a mature adult, you will have a natural sensational performance level. When entering the sexual arena with your spouse, always be sure to leave your role of mom and child-minder behind and be in your mature adult mindset. This is the moment which God has given you and you are allowed to enjoy it!

When your marriage is mature in faith, it is good to know intimacy starts with praying together and loving God first. It is encouraging to see your husband reading his Bible and praying for God to protect you and your children, or putting the children to bed and praying for them. Your femininity will grow stronger when you see your husband so strong, powerful and such a giant in the world, being humble, gentle and loving with God, you and the children. This spiritual security can be very romantic and intimate, and make you feel safe.

Because Jesus Christ has set you free, you have an advantage in your marriage to be the best you can be. Buy yourself sexy lingerie and let it be a secret between you and your husband. You can even give the lingerie names like avalanche or pink flamingo to make it fun, and then send each other messages about the lingerie while you have a tea break at work!

Here are some ideas to spice up your sex life. When you and your husband are alone for the weekend, have sex with your most expensive high heels on, for no particular reason, just because it is different. Have sex in the kitchen on the counter top; the chill of the counter should bring great excitement to the sex act and the counter top will lift you to his level if he is slightly taller than you. Have wet sex with your husband; do not dry yourself after taking a bath or shower. You might like it just because it is different. When you are in the mood for sex, run to the room while undressing, running like you want to get caught and if he does not notice (he is, after all, a man!) ask him to catch you; or be a bit of a tease. The youthfulness in you can be a great turn-on. If you are overweight and shy about it, make a decision to enjoy taking your clothes off and making love to your husband even while the light is on. Some men enjoy the change and you do not have to worry much about moving forwards and backwards, up or down. Moving your buttocks in circles is a winner and does not leave you breathless.

We cannot agree more about weight being an important health matter, but let it stay in the department of health, not in the department of sexual intercourse, not in the department of fashion and not in the department of relationships. If the thought of your weight stops you from taking off your clothes or wearing something sexy for your spouse, put it back in the department where it belongs!

Memories are wonderful to take with you to your old age, so make your sexual adventures a lifetime of great memories. You can never be too old to be the best you can be, and it is always good to leave space in your life for change. You might think your husband will not like a change, but surprise him! People grow older, they learn things and their needs change, even in the bedroom. Sex gets better when you grow older. This was confirmed by a couple of 70 years old!

Are you and your husband living fulfilled sexual lives? It is an intimate and important part of the marriage rarely spoken about. The only way to be sure whether your spouse is content with your marriage is to find out by asking. Ask him when you are both relaxed and in a private place whether there is anything he would like to try out or even like to think about trying. Tell him what your fantasies are and try to make them a reality.

Talk to your husband about a few things you would like to try, whether they are different positions or a different place to make love or approaching sex in a different way. If you do not feel like accommodating your husband with a suggestion he makes, you have the right to say so, but think about it before refusing; you may feel the need to accommodate him and vice versa. Remember, suggestions have a tendency not always to work out the first time; so be ready to fail miserably at it, have a good laugh, make love in a way you are both familiar with, and then try again some other time. Have fun. Sex is supposed to be fun and enjoyable!

Sex is not only a physical experience, but an emotional and spiritual experience as well. Approach sexual intercourse with the Holy Spirit's guidance and even allow Him to give you some sexual direction and ideas on what to try and experiment with in the bedroom. Never leave God out of your sex life; He is God of all of you, whether you are having sex, fighting, hurting or laughing.

Never make emotionally directed decisions. You cannot live according to your emotions or feelings. Make decisions according to the Word of God under the guidance of the Holy Spirit. It sometimes feels as if the world is about to cave in on you; this is normal and everyone goes through this. Separate yourself from the situation causing you the unnecessary stress and tension and deal with it in prayer; only then make an active and realistic decision before moving on.

Thought capturing is a fantastic way to deal with controlling emotions in order to gain perspective on life, your situation and circumstances again. What is thought capturing? It is a simple process. Listen to the thought you are having, realise what it is about and say to God, 'Lord, I submit this thought to you, please help me to distinguish between my feelings and what You are saying through the Holy Spirit and Your Word. I take my thoughts captive and make them subject to Yours and pray that you will bless my thoughts in the Name of Jesus. Amen!' You may say your own prayer; this is merely a suggestion.

6.3 Sex toys

Sex toys can be incorporated when one spouse is temporarily or permanently unable to use their genitals for sexual intercourse or when sexual dysfunction is present. It is every couple's decision whether they want to incorporate sexual toys in their marriage bed or not. Sex toys are sometimes also incorporated in healthy marriages as part of foreplay or even sometimes just to bring variety into the bedroom.

If and when your sexual status returns to normal, pursue natural sexual intercourse again. Sex toys are never to replace natural sexual intercourse, but only to assist and complement it.

When using sex toys ensure there is enough lubrication in order not to cause injury. If natural lubrication is a problem, you may purchase water-based lubricant gel to supplement lubrication. Please do not put water in the vagina in an attempt to lubricate as this is unhealthy and can be dangerous.

6.4 Vibrators

Vibrators are designed for different purposes. Clitoral vibrators are sometimes also massaging vibrators; they were created to stimulate the nerve ends on the body and to release relaxing hormones. Vaginal vibrators are shaped to stimulate the G-spot or clitoris. Do not attempt to use a vaginal vibrator as an anal vibrator as it is not shaped for anal use and could cause injury to your spouse.

To enjoy vibrators within your marriage together with your spouse, you need some practise. Spend some time planning and enjoying it, being focussed on intimacy and romance and mutual sexual satisfaction rather than being self-indulgent.

In the same way that you drive a vehicle in a good or a bad way, you can also use a sex toy either for the benefit of your Kingdom marriage or to benefit your selfish desires. Should the latter be your intention, it is time for you to be honest with yourself and your spouse and fix the problem. The best way to find out whether it is time for the sex toy to be put away is to watch your spouse's expression while you are making use of it. A positive or negative reaction should be a clear indication whether it is wise to continue using the toy or not.

When making use of a vibrator, do not have a belittling attitude towards yourself or your spouse. Treat your body and your spouse's body with love, compassion and respect.

Do not allow a vibrator to become an extramarital affair you are having with modern technology. It may result in your spouse becoming jealous of the toy and it may lead to feelings of incompetence. Always use a vibrator as a help tool and never as a replacement tool.

Every spouse using a vibrator has their own style, but some basic suggestions on how to use it may be mentioned. You need to be in a relaxed, private atmosphere knowing you have enough time. First rub your genitals and surrounding areas with your hands, also stimulating other sensitive areas on your body. Switch your vibrator on and gently glide it over your skin where you rubbed with your hands, but not on your clitoris yet. The best way is to involve your spouse in the process.

Take time to enjoy the moment, then move to your vagina and back up to your clitoris. Concentrate on stimulating the surrounding areas more than your clitoris, occasionally penetrating the vagina, then to the clitoris, but not so that you climax, and then back to the vagina. Rotate this action while using your other hand to massage parts of your body, feeling how wonderfully you are made and what sensations you arouse.

Slip the vibrator into the vagina, moving firmly and more rapidly, again rotating between the vagina and clitoris, and when your clitoris is properly excited, hold the vibrator to it until you climax. Slide it back into your vagina and penetrate until you climax with the vibrator against your G-spot. This is just a basic suggestion; you may develop your own style or even change the style you have. Allow your husband to touch you while you are using the vibrator or even let him use the vibrator on you, but you will have to guide him so he does not over stimulate, causing you discomfort. This is an excellent way for you to grow the trust between you and your spouse, also practising open sexual communication.

Be careful that you do not compare vibrators with what you experience with natural sexual intercourse. They are two totally different things and you should enjoy each experience for what it is.

6.5 Condoms

Different variations of condoms are on the market and they are usually found in supermarkets closest to the counters. There are coloured ones, different shaped ones, different sizes and differently flavoured condoms. You may want to keep condoms around for the purpose of exploring, protection or birth control.

Cover the erect penis with the condom. To ensure safety remember to change it immediately once you have climaxed or if it breaks or tears. Remove and discard it before you next have intercourse.

As a married couple, it is your choice whether you want to use condoms or not.

Female condoms are freely available everywhere, but are not as commonly used, and are very effective. You can obtain them from your nearest family planning institution, clinic or hospital.

Condoms do lessen sensitivity for the husband, making them good products to use when he struggles with premature ejaculation. They may help him to last longer, keep his erection longer and be able to learn how to control his ejaculation.

6.6 Other

There are various other things that can be used during sex and foreplay and as long as these contribute to your sex life and they are not inspired by lust, enjoy making them part of your marriage. Feathers can be used to gently stroke your spouse's body during foreplay. Balloons can be filled with lukewarm to cool water and rubbed on the genitals or the body. You can use lubrication on the balloon but never use balloons internally. Chocolate body paint is very attractive, as long as your spouse can appreciate being sticky. Chocolate body paint can be used to stimulate both spouse's nipples, inner thigh areas and anywhere else on the body by smearing it on and slowly eating it off. Honey can be used for the same purpose as well as ice, should your spouse agree. Edible underwear can be incredibly attractive and mysterious because it is not commonly used.

Discuss edible lingerie with your spouse and find out whether it should be part of your sex life. Whenever you use a homemade product, please always consider safety first.

6.7 Summary

Born again believers are free through the Lord, Jesus Christ, who died for all sins and rose again on the third day to overcome death and is now at the right hand of God in heaven.

Being teachable within the safe boundaries of your marriage, under the guidance of the Holy Spirit and the Bible, will encourage the curious, playful person you are. You have been given your specific circumstances to overcome, to enjoy, to live to the glory of your Father in heaven and to be blessed accordingly.

God created you as either male or female and you should be comfortable with the gender you are while loving your spouse for being the opposite gender. Never allow gender to become an issue preventing you from having sex. Embrace your gender, enjoy who you are and realise your spouse has been created differently for a purpose; to complete you.

Men and women have been created very differently; not only physically, but emotionally, spiritually, socially and sexually. Understanding the fact that men think about sex constantly and are always and immediately ready for sex just by smelling or seeing or being near their wives will make wives have more consideration for the way their husbands have been created. When men understand their wives are made very differently and that it usually takes time for them to get ready for sex, it will cause husbands to be creative in turning their wives on regularly and constantly. Sex is a physical experience for men; something enjoyable to pass time and release sexual tension. For women, however, sex is a 'complete personal involvement' experience and they want to truly be loved by their husbands and feel good about their spouses and themselves before they can really let go and give over to the enjoyment of sexual intercourse.

These differences should be taken in to consideration during sex and husbands should spend time helping their wives reach orgasm even if they have already ejaculated. It is always recommended that the husband let his wife reach orgasm at the same time as his own ejaculation or before, because after ejaculation the penis usually loses erection and it will be difficult for his wife to reach orgasm. If he ejaculated before his wife reached orgasm, the husband should actively and enthusiastically help his wife to reach orgasm and release tension in any way possible; moving the penis over the clitoris, manual stimulation, oral sex, masturbation or making use of a sex toy.

Sex toys should be used to assist in sexual intercourse and never as a replacement for natural sexual intercourse.

Sex is created to be enjoyed. If you embrace your gender while considering your spouse's gender and purposefully pursue enjoyable sex, you will fulfil your desires in a whole new adventure.

CHAPTER 7

Third party

Bringing a third party into your marriage is the first step towards marital disaster, leading to numerous problems and deep seated unhappiness for both you and your spouse.

Involving a third person in your marriage is a sign that something is wrong in your marriage or between you and your spouse. A third party would never be involved in your marriage if everything else in your life and marriage was fine.

There are numerous ways a third person is able to infiltrate your marriage, but it is always preceded by unhappiness or one of the spouses not getting what he or she should be getting or expects to be getting from the marriage relationship. This is not an excuse to allow a third person into the marriage, but a reason why it happens.

It is not difficult to invite a third person into your marriage, but it always leads to immeasurable heartache and problems afterwards. It takes a real man to keep his wife happy for the rest of their lives and it takes a real woman to keep her husband happy for the rest of their lives. It is easy to have extra-marital sex but it is not the biblical way and it is certainly not the path to a successful marriage.

Your responsibility in your marriage is two-fold; firstly, you are responsible for your own happiness within your marriage, and secondly, it is your responsibility to make your spouse want you, while at the same time bringing out the inner passion in yourself and in your spouse. Living this way will eliminate the need for a third person in your marriage, resulting in a fulfilled marriage characterised by unleashed inner sexual passion in you and your spouse.

Marriage is a gift from God so allowing a third party into your marriage relationship is a sure way of showing God exactly how little you think of the gift He has given you. Seeing your marriage as a gift also places a huge responsibility on you to make the most of it. You should work at your marriage to ensure both your own and your spouse's happiness while actively keeping any third party away.

Marriage should be kept exclusive and your wedding bed should be kept undefiled from any third party to ensure purity, but what happens if a third party has crept into your marriage? Do you simply file for divorce or do you work on the marriage? Adultery is a valid biblical reason to get a divorce,[51] but just because it is a legitimate reason, it does not have to end up as such. You may make the decision to work on your marriage instead of giving up, but ultimately the choice is yours and it will take a lot from you to forgive your spouse.

Maybe you are the guilty spouse or maybe you are the innocent one, but you should be fully aware of the dangers of a third party entering your marriage and the resulting consequences.

7.1 Third party variations

Inviting a third person into your marriage can take on many forms, but regardless of the manner the results are always devastating. The way in which a third person accesses your marriage is irrelevant when viewed from a biblical perspective, because it is still seen as adultery and not acceptable in the sight of God.

Involving a third person in a marriage can be based either on sex only, or it can be mainly emotional in nature, or it can be a combination of sex and emotions. Involvement of the third party usually begins either around sex or talking about the problems experienced in the marriage. The relationship with the third person is usually very one-sided.

Maybe you are the third party reading this book and if so, we have only one question for you: Are you not worth more and do you not deserve more than to be the third person in a relationship?

7.1.1 One-night stand

The so-called one-night stand is when you casually meet someone and you are both so filled with lust that neither of you even try to resist the urge to have sex. Usually this person is a stranger and you might not even know his or her name.

The one-night stand is based purely on sex and, more accurately, lust! One of the dangers of one-night stands is that you do not know what sexually transmitted diseases the person may be carrying. You also do not know the person's background so the risks are high.

Getting involved in a one-night stand actually says much more about the spouse who messes up in this way than of the third person. If the spouse is willing to throw everything away for someone unknown based purely on lust, it is a sign of utter immaturity and disregard for the marriage. Spending time evaluating why you are willing to place your marriage in jeopardy will hopefully bring an answer about where the root problem in the marriage lies.

7.1.2 Prostitution

Prostitution is when someone is paid for sex and it is just as bad as the one-night stand and in some instances actually much worse. What makes prostitution worse than the one-night stand is that the prostitute is much more susceptible to sexually transmitted diseases.

The question should be asked why a married person would even consider paying a total stranger for sex. Is it because you are not getting sex in your marriage or is it because of lust and wanting too much sex, resulting in your spouse being unable to keep up? Is the need for sex with a prostitute based on wanting to have sex with more than one person or wanting to unleash an inner sexual passion but being too scared to discuss it with your spouse?

Whatever the reason, visiting a prostitute is definitely not the solution. Discuss your needs openly with your spouse instead of bringing a third person into your marriage in the form of a prostitute.

7.1.3 Affair

A full-fledged affair is usually about more than just sex. An affair is when you get emotionally and sexually involved with someone other than your spouse, and spend time together as if you were a couple. Often the person you are having an affair with is also married.

Affairs usually involve lots of sex as well as sexual experimentation, but they are normally not the result of a need for sex. Affairs are generally started because of the marital problems of both people involved in the affair. Conversations in affairs more often than not evolve around the topic of sex, but avoid the actual subject of why the affair began in the first place.

Having an affair is a way of not dealing with your marital problems, but rather running away from them. An affair will never be the solution to the problems; it will just end up adding further problems to a marriage already experiencing problems.

What makes affairs so dangerous is the emotional involvement and the consequences. Often two people having an affair become so involved with each other that they are willing to get divorced from their spouses, leading to families getting hurt in the process. The worst part, however, is when these two people actually get divorced from their spouses and then enter into a relationship or even marriage with each other, but are then unable to find fulfilment because their relationship is not based on trust; they live in fear of losing their new partner because if the partner could cheat on their spouse, he or she may also cheat on you.

This is a real concern and something to consider before embarking on an affair.

7.1.4 Polygamy

Polygamy is when someone is married to more than one spouse with or without the knowledge of all the spouses involved.

In Western culture polygamy is a criminal offence and it is usually without the spouses' knowledge. In other words, someone might marry two or more spouses without them knowing about each other. In Western culture, this is usually done by someone who travels a lot and has different spouses in different cities.

This form of polygamy is mostly due to two reasons; firstly because of loneliness as a result of travelling extensively and being away from a spouse regularly, and secondly due to the need for having sex with more than one person.

In certain cultures polygamy is an accepted practice in which the various spouses are aware of each other and sometimes even live together in the same house. In these cultures it is usually one man that has numerous wives, but never the other way around. We should consider why these cultures allow polygamy. Does the man think it is his right to have sex with different women on a regular basis and has a way to do it acceptably within his culture? Polygamy is clearly wrong according to the Bible; read 1 Corinthians 7:2 and Ephesians 5:33 as good examples.

Whatever the reasons behind polygamy, it always leads to spouses feeling they are not good enough to satisfy their spouse's sexual needs. If you are part of a polygamous relationship, think about why you want to be part of such a group and the answer to this question may highlight what issues need attention in your life.

7.1.5 Threesome

Threesomes involve a third person in your marriage bed, in other words, three people having sex together. Depending on the married couple, either a man or a woman is invited into the bed.

The reasons why threesomes are usually brought into a marriage are because of lust and for 'spicing up' the marital relationship. Threesomes are seen as a way to get more excitement into the marriage bed, but what is never taken into account is what the effects will be when the third person leaves.

After a threesome has taken place, one of the spouses almost always feels inadequate to sexually satisfy their spouse and that the threesome was necessary to achieve what he or she was unable to. The gender of the third person will also have a major influence on how the married couple reacts afterwards; usually it is the spouse of the same gender as the third person who will feel like this. Threesomes are dangerous in that it will set a precedent in the marriage and the longing will always be there to do it again 'because it has been done already'.

7.1.6 Swinging

Swinging is the practice of two married couples swapping spouses in order to have sex with the other couple's spouse. This is done either in private or in an orgy-type environment where both couples are in one room.

Just like threesomes, swinging is also based on lust and for 'spicing up' the marriage. Swinging does not spice up the marriage, but rather brings problems into it. More often than not swinging starts off as a once-off sexual experiment but ends up with one of the spouses becoming involved in an affair with a spouse from the other married couple. Whether it ends up in an affair or not, swinging is still dangerous and not only because of sexually transmitted diseases, but also because the subconscious message being sent to your spouse is a message of sexual incompetence and the inability to satisfy you.

7.1.7 Foursome

Foursomes are when another couple is invited into the bedroom and then the two couples have sex in the presence of one another. In a foursome, each couple only has sex with their own partners or spouses, but it is done in the presence of the other couple. In other words, the two couples have sex with their own spouses in the same room as the other couple.

Even though sex with a third party is not actually taking place, this is seen as involving a third party in your marriage. Foursomes are not healthy because once again the subconscious message to your spouse is that your spouse is not good enough to satisfy your needs. Consider why you have the need to have sex in front of another couple.

7.1.8 Sexual addiction

Sexual addiction should be mentioned due to the enormous negative effect it has not only on a marriage relationship, but also with the relationship such a person has with himself or herself. People struggling with sexual addiction will have sex with anyone or anything just to experience the feeling of sexual release in an attempt to feel good.

People with a sexual addiction usually have low self-images and having sex with as many people they can actually worsens the low self-image, causing the person to enter a vicious cycle of feeling worse and worse about him-or-herself. Sexual addiction is often a crutch used to escape some negative circumstance or situation in life and not wanting to deal with it appropriately.

Sexual addiction is just as bad as any other form of addiction or even worse. If a married person is addicted to sex it does not only cause problems in the marriage due to involving third parties, but it also makes the fear of sexually transmitted diseases a reality for the innocent spouse. Sexual addiction is seldom about sex, but usually about the underlying problem.

We have talked about the various ways of involving a third party in your marriage and they all can be seen as adultery clearly forbidden by God Himself, but why do spouses become involved in extramarital sex? The Bible gives a good indication in Romans 1:24-28 of why people sometimes get involved in extramarital sex, but based on Romans 1:7, where Christians are called to live a consecrated life unto God and choosing not to, may lead to adultery. So let us look at why spouses commit adultery from a human perspective.

7.2 Why do spouses commit adultery?

Excuses given for committing adultery are usually based on blaming a spouse for not fulfilling all your sexual needs or never being there or because of not taking responsibility for the state your marriage is in.

But usually adultery is committed because of allowing impure thoughts into your mind instead of working on your marriage to find sexual fulfilment with your spouse. Blame is often put on the spouse for not fulfilling all your needs and wants in the marriage, but each person should take responsibility for their own lives and actions, regardless of their spouse's behaviour. This can reach a point where a spouse just does not care anymore and when such a point is reached, adultery might occur without the person even having second thoughts about it.

Adultery is mostly the result of unhappiness in the marriage and the inability to effectively communicate this feeling to the spouse. People deciding to commit adultery often feel it is their right to do so, because their spouse did not make any effort to change when the problem was discussed. What every person should realise is that their own actions and decisions are based on their attitude and not on the spouse's actions. You should take full responsibility for your own actions and decisions and live with the consequences. What should be remembered is the One you will have to answer to for committing adultery is ultimately not your spouse, but God Himself.

Sexual experimentation is another reason for committing adultery. If one spouse does not want to sexually experiment and try out new things and new sexual positions, the other spouse may think it is good enough reason to commit adultery so that he or she can experiment. This is the wrong approach, however, and instead of spending all the time and money on a third party, why not spend the same amount of time, money and energy in loving your spouse? You might be surprised at how open he or she will become in trying new things. Your spouse will realise that he or she and your marriage are very important to you and then more of an effort and willingness to experiment may be the result.

One of the most common reasons for committing adultery is when a person is mad at God and wants to get back at Him, using adultery as the means of doing it. This is a very risky method of trying to get back at God and will not only result in your spiritual life being hurt tremendously, but also in your spouse being hurt and your marriage entering dangerous ground.

7.3 Warning signs of adultery

Adultery is not always easy to spot because the spouse committing adultery is usually very careful not to be caught. Regardless of how careful the person is, there are always warning signs indicating the possibility that adultery is being committed.

Dishonesty is usually a first sign. If your spouse is dishonest and lies about small things, it may indicate that your spouse is also willing to lie and be dishonest about bigger things like committing adultery. Dishonesty could be a characteristic of your spouse and you would know whether lying is an issue for him or her or rather a lifestyle.

When your spouse spends lots of time away from you, it should be seen as a warning sign. It may be due to spending time with a third party. Spending unusual amounts of time on the telephone or on the Internet may also be warning signs, especially when your spouse does not want you nearby when making the calls or surfing the Internet. When a spouse regularly goes on business trips, it might be another warning sign. Being aware of other warning signs is therefore important.

One of the main warning sign for unfaithfulness is when your spouse constantly compares you to other people and is degrading to you or your sexual ability. Be aware of comments like 'My friend's spouse allows this or that in the bedroom, why do you not want to even consider it?' This type of remark should be a warning to you, not of your spouse having already committed adultery, but for you to become aware that adultery is becoming a reality in your spouse's mind because you are unwilling to experiment in your sexual relationship.

Another warning sign is when your spouse repeatedly arrives home late, using the excuse of having to work late. It obviously depends on your spouse's career and there might be good reason to work late, but how sure are you that your spouse is working late?

Overall unhappiness with your sexual relationship and marriage is another possible cause for adultery. If your spouse is unhappy all the time and not willing to do anything about it, the possibility of adultery may be running around in your spouse's mind or maybe it has even gone further already.

There are other warning signs for adultery, but you should always remember to give your spouse the benefit of the doubt. Never suspect your spouse of having committed adultery because one of the warning signs are present, but always view a warning sign as a signal for you to invest more time in your marriage and sexual relationship so as to ensure your marriage is strong and able to resist any temptations from third parties.

If you and your spouse are happily married and sexually fulfilled, you will not even be tempted when placed in a situation where a third party makes a move. Not flirting and not entertaining the thought of committing adultery and having sex with this third party is a sure sign of a marriage in excellent shape, without adultery even being a possibility. Spend time making your marriage the happy relationship it can be and ensure your spouse has an unleashed inner passion based on marital sexual fulfilment.

7.4 Effects of adultery

The effects of adultery are always based on hurt and pain while being characterised by broken relationships and inner heartache.

Adultery is never easy to deal with, because it is always a subconscious sign of sexual incompetence and the inability to be a good spouse. Adultery always portrays the subliminal message of not being good enough and not worth the effort to make the marriage work. Adultery is like a slap in the face, saying you are worthless and not worth staying pure for. Adultery also says the marriage vows taken before God are not worth protecting and ultimately you are not worth protection or even the effort of trying.

It is not difficult to realise how devastating it is for someone to come to terms with a spouse having committed adultery. It is always accompanied by hurt, pain, fear and negative feelings of worthlessness and incompetence.

On the other hand, maybe you are the one who committed adultery and these are the messages you sent to your spouse, hurting your spouse tremendously in the process. You might realise it was not worth it, but you do not know what to do to correct the hurt and pain you caused. You may want to work on your marriage, but it is not up to you; your spouse should make the decision whether to be willing to work on the marriage or not.

If your spouse wants to rather get a divorce, you may try and persuade him or her not to, but ultimately you do not have a say as you were the one who committed adultery and hurt your spouse in the process. Decide to give your spouse the necessary space to make the decision that will work for him or her, and then accept the decision without making it more difficult for your spouse than it already is.

7.5 How to correct the effects of adultery

Correcting the effects of adultery is not always possible and the hurt and pain might be so deep-seated nothing can be done to correct it. In this instance the marriage will most probably end up in a divorce and the person who committed adultery will have the divorce and marriage failure on his or her conscience.

Whether the marriage goes the divorce route or whether the decision is taken to work on the marriage and try to work out the problems, it all will have to start with the guilty party asking forgiveness and the innocent party fully granting forgiveness. It should start with asking forgiveness from God and then from the spouse, and in return forgiveness should be given to the guilty spouse because of Him, and for the innocent spouse's sanity and future. Forgiveness may be a process, but if the couple is willing to go on the journey and walk through the process, it will be possible to fully forgive and work on the marriage without any resentment.

It should also be said that the effects of adultery can only be corrected if both spouses go to God with the problem, and possibly to a good marriage counsellor, while firstly working on their spiritual lives and secondly on their marriage. Openly communicate about the reasons why the adultery occurred and then something practical should be done about the causes of the adultery. Without dealing with and eliminating the causes of adultery, it is possible that it may re-occur later.

Correcting the effects of adultery may be a daunting task and a long process of healing and rebuilding trust again, but it is a journey worth embarking on and definitely worth the effort.

7.6 Spiritual healing after adultery

Adultery will always have a negative affect on your spiritual life and your relationship with God, regardless of why you committed adultery. God cannot bless you and pour out his favour upon you if you are living in sin, and committing adultery is a lifestyle of sin that you chose to enter into.

There is never an excuse for it. Adultery is always the result of a choice made, and the first step towards spiritual healing after adultery is to take full responsibility for all the actions and decisions you made. If you have committed adultery, take responsibility, acknowledge it and confess your sin to God. If you are the innocent party, take responsibility for your part in the unhappy marriage, which may have lead to your spouse committing adultery.

After confessing your sin and taking responsibility for your mistakes, you need to forgive; Firstly forgive God. This might sound ridiculous, but it might be necessary to forgive God even though He did not cause your spouse to commit adultery; you might have been blaming Him for it and therefore you need to 'forgive' God by releasing Him from all responsibility for what your spouse has done to you. Forgive yourself, forgive your spouse and forgive the third party. Even if you are the innocent party, you must forgive. The benefits of forgiveness are never for anyone else, but always for you personally; when you release the guilty parties to God, you are separating yourself from the punishment because it is not your responsibility to punish or judge anyone.

God is the only one able to truly heal you spiritually after adultery and therefore you should seek Him daily. Try to restore your spiritual life by spending time with Him and allowing Him to lead and guide you again. This will lead to you being healed spiritually one day at a time. God is able to heal you in one touch, but spiritual healing after adultery is usually a process of healing combined with laying down bad habits and picking up new and healthy habits.

A good Christian marriage counsellor will be of great value to you during this process of spiritual healing, but also as someone you can be accountable towards for your actions in the days to come.

7.7 Soul ties

When two people have sexual intercourse they become one flesh[52] and that means a special bond is created between them; in other words, a soul tie develops between them.

A soul tie is a bond or emotional connection between people and sexual intercourse is not the only way it can occur, but it is one of the ways. Sex was intended for married people to be linked to each other when two individuals become one in marriage.

When a spouse committs adultery, such a soul tie is formed with a third person. Because it is unhealthy to be connected to someone other than your spouse, such a soul tie should be broken.

Breaking a soul tie can only occur when the sin has been confessed, forgiveness has been extended to those involved and when you are really willing to break all ties with the third person to such an extent as to never see the person or even talk to the person again. When this foundation has been laid, breaking a soul tie can be done with a prayer like:

Lord, I renounce this unhealthy union with the third person based on what I have done, and I ask you to break this soul tie connection between us completely and set us free from each other.

7.8 Marital sex after adultery

After adultery has occurred and you and your spouse decided to work on your marriage rather than getting a divorce, the very important matter of marital sex will arise between you and your spouse. How will you deal with sex again? Will the adultery always be a barrier between the two of you, preventing you from truly enjoying marital sex again?

Marital sex after adultery is one of the most difficult acts for the innocent spouse in the marriage, because thoughts of the guilty spouse with the third party will constantly be an obstacle. It can be overcome, however, if there is true forgiveness and a real dedication to making the marriage work.

A first step would be for both spouses to go for testing to ensure there are no sexually transmitted diseases. With adultery comes the increased possibility of transferring a sexually transmitted disease to an innocent spouse, and consequently health tests should be completed to ensure safety in this area.

Marital sex after adultery can sometimes be better than before, especially if it is accompanied by dedication from both spouses to really make it work while eliminating the reasons for why the adultery originally occurred. Marital sex after adultery can become a platform for your inner sexual passion and your spouse's to be unleashed, and it is possible to find true sexual fulfilment in your marriage once again or maybe for the first time.

7.9 Summary

Adultery is never easy to overcome, but if there is true dedication and a commitment to making the marriage work, it can be overcome successfully without it ever becoming an obstacle or a temptation again. Both spouses need to make a one hundred percent commitment to making the marriage work and to building the marriage on a biblical foundation, as well as biblical principles.

Adultery may occur in many forms, but whatever form it comes in and regardless of whether it happens with the spouse's knowledge or permission or not, it is still adultery and God sees it as such. As a Christian married couple you should want to make God smile on your marriage and do what He requires of you, namely to stay clear of all forms of adultery without exception. Stay committed to your spouse and keep yourselves clean within the boundaries of your marriage.

If you are the innocent party, you must make the decision whether to stay with your spouse and make your marriage work or to get a divorce. Whatever you decide must be a biblical decision, because God does not like divorce, but Jesus said adultery is a valid reason to get a divorce. Your decision will be something you will have to live with for the rest of your life, so take your time in making the correct decision.

If you decide to stay with your spouse, work together to eliminate the reasons the adultery occurred in the first place and openly communicate about the problems in your marriage so they can be dealt with effectively. If you think it will be impossible to deal with this on your own, do not hesitate to call in the help of a professional, but ensure this professional is supporting your Christian faith and beliefs about marriage. Also remember you will have to engage in sexual intercourse with your spouse again and if you have truly forgiven your spouse and are able to do this, you should provide the platform within your marriage for some sexual experimentation and the unleashing of your inner sexual passion as well as your spouse's in order for true sexual fulfilment to enter your marriage.

If you are the guilty party who committed adultery, confess your sin and ask for forgiveness, then turn your back on the past and move on without ever even considering falling for the temptation of adultery and extramarital sex again. In future, avoid any situation where there might even be the slightest possibility of being tempted in this way again. Openly communicate with your spouse about your needs and wants while dealing with the root causes of why you entered into the adulterous relationship in the first place. Your biggest challenge will be to put open communication in place instead of keeping everything under wraps, then acting out in the form of adultery. This immature behaviour should be eliminated.

Adultery is sin in the eyes of God and it is always accompanied by spiritual decay, tremendous hurt, pain and fear, but there is life after adultery. If you are willing to confess your sin and turn your back on the sin of adultery, you will be able to continue with your life.

God is a God of love and He is willing to forgive you totally if you confess your sin and repent; that is, turning your back on the sin and never to doing it again. You can put adultery behind you, but then you must also keep your mind pure and clean, not allowing any impure thoughts to enter your mind because adultery is not only the sexual act, but also the thought of the sexual act with anyone other than your spouse.

CHAPTER 8

Turn-ons and turn-offs

8.1 What are sexual turn-offs?

The single most terrible sexual turn-off is sin. No one wants to be lied to, deceived, mistrusted, suspected, judged, underestimated, controlled, manipulated, abused, disrespected or mistreated, sworn at, rebuked, hated or forced to do or accept anything.

Never allow yourself or your spouse to engage in a belittling sexual action. It is vital that you respect your body and your spouse's body. Should you have had such an encounter, it is important to repair it. Forgiveness and renewed respect should be the end result of such action. If it seems impossible to repair, then you need to pray. Belittling actions are not from the kingdom of God and should never be entertained at any time or for any reason.

Any addictions are a major turn-off since they kill intimacy, the very glue of God's grace and mercy for sexual intercourse. The purest form of making love is being pure while making love. Let me repeat this: the purest form of making love is being pure while making love. It is something worth achieving and most definitely possible since Jesus Christ died for your sins and rose again on the third day. The meaning of being pure does not mean being perfect. Being pure means accepting that Jesus Christ died for your bad side while striving to live out your good side with the help of the Holy Spirit.

Sexual interactions are not counselling sessions. Do not talk about anything offensive or worrisome while engaging in sex. Focus on the sexual encounter and enjoy the moment while putting all worries outside the door.

More sexual turn-offs include bad body odours, poor hygiene, poor body language, insecurity, engaging sexually but not really being fully committed, selfishness, bad sexual experiences, pride, poor moral values, poor manners, sarcasm, negative attitudes from the husband or the wife, and sickness. Purposefully being bombastic, spiteful or revengeful is a definite turn-off for any spouse. Where there is no love, kindness, care, compassion, hope, faith, knowledge or wisdom you can be sure that your partner will be turned-off.

Fear is a sexual turn-off. Having a fight, being belittled and being manipulated into sex is never a turn-on and should always be avoided. Focusing your attention on things other than sexuality while your spouse may be aroused is a turn-off.

Do not force your spouse to pray with you before or after engaging sexually. The Christian faith is not a forced act. At any time when something is forced upon a person, their enthusiasm, creativity, excitement and courage are strained. Their freedom is limited which is just as good as non-existent. True Christianity will result in spouses wanting to pray together without having to be forced to do so.

Even while being in sin, every person has the right to overcome it in their own time, so let them as it gives a foundation for positive personal growth. You may ask, 'How is your progress in overcoming the situation or problem?' or 'Always know that when you need my help, I am right here for you and we can pray about it together'. This is much better than preaching to your spouse. Instead loving your spouse back to being the person you know he or she can be.

8.2 What are sexual turn-ons?

The five senses play a role in sexual turn-ons, but what is sexually exciting for one spouse is not necessarily a turn-on for the other. Let's look at some sexual turn-ons.

What you hear. Have you ever tuned your ears to your spouse's voice, the kindness as they speak and the lovely things they say? Listen to them when they say something nice to you or comment positively or simply agree or even laugh or whisper. Your spouse's voice could lead to a great sexual turn-on. Other auditory turn-ons could be listening to music together, the breathing of your spouse, their heartbeat or kisses, moaning or vocal exclamations of love, even touching and massaging the ears, nibbling the lobes or stroking the top of the ears. Some couples like confirming their love for each other while making love by saying how much they love each other. Apparently eating apples is a very sexual sound. You can try this as a sexual turn-on.

What you see. Looking at your spouse, seeing how they behave, dress, react and what their loving body language is, is a very important part of your marriage. Your attitude resulting from positive thoughts towards your spouse speaks louder than words. Putting the Word of God into action will help you to develop a positive attitude by focusing on what you have instead of what you do not have. Create a pleasant visual of something relaxing and calming to look at, such as candles, soft materials, dimmed light, romantic venues, rose petals and a bathtub filled with bubbles. Your spouse wants to see a loving, kind facial expression, even while having sex. Wearing white clothes, see-through clothes or absolutely nothing while alone with your spouse can also be a great turn-on.

One of the biggest sexual turn-ons is self-confidence, but not when you are consumed with yourself all the time; rather where you know you are good, and you can show it to your spouse with a smile.

Some husbands and wives like their spouses to be suggestive and teasing, rather than inviting and available, or vice versa. You can try these to see what you both prefer.

Sex is a pleasurable act and it is sexy to see your spouse enjoying themselves. Looking at your spouse enjoying sex is a huge turn-on.

Create great visual turn-ons for your spouse, for example, his or her own private strip show, dancing in a seductive manner, creating sensational body language and not moving too fast. It is not just important to see how wonderful God made your spouse, but also to allow your spouse to look at you as well, so allow him or her to take in the detail of your movements.

Looking at your spouse or your spouse looking at you while you are naked can be a great turn-on. Openly discuss this with your spouse in advance because private individuals may find this offensive even when practiced within the safe boundaries of marriage.

What you smell and taste. The smell of perfume, deodorant, certain foods, your spouse's skin, fresh air, clean breath and homely smells are all important sexual turn-ons. You may not even notice it, but your smelling sense picks up the need of your spouse to be loved. Body smells are released when you become sexually turned-on. Do not hide this with too much perfume or deodorant. You will find it is very sexy and it creates great sexual pleasure. Smelling your spouse's skin and body will assist in creating intimacy. It could create an intense closeness. The taste of your spouse's lips, tongue, sucking the fingers, or licking the skin and genitals could be a great turn-on for you both. Taste is intimate because it is wet and there are several taste buds on the tongue. Combine tasting with a gentle sucking, nibbling, blowing and kissing to sensitive areas of the skin, for instance, the neck, nipples and some spouses may even like their toes sucked!

What you touch and feel. The lips are very sensitive. You might want to rub your fingers (not tickle) across your spouse's lips or kiss them. Exploring your spouse's body with your mouth can be a great sexual turn-on.

Touching your spouse by stroking, rubbing or hugging can send electric feelings up and down their spine. As sexual tension intensifies between you, your touch can become firmer rather than simply stroking and cuddling. Sexual tension does not have to fade between you and your spouse over time. You can be sexy at any time for your spouse and an unexpected kiss or sexual advance at the right time can cause an incredible sexual turn-on for you both. People need to feel wanted and knowing your spouse wants you is sexually inviting.

When, however, sexual tension has become a problem, you need to change your own mind about the way you view the sexual side of your spouse.

Holding hands might be an old-fashioned way of connecting intimately, but it always works, especially when the tension of love is electrified between the two of you and the hand is lightly squeezed or held firmly, and then followed by a French kiss or complete silence.

What you taste and touch with your mouth. The mouth is an effective erotic instrument with several sensational qualities. Your smile can be a huge turn-on as well as the way you eat, speak or say romantic things. Blowing a kiss, licking your lips and the way you bite your lips may be very sexy to your spouse. Kissing your spouse's body and tasting your spouse's lips, tongue and body is a turn-on, just like whispering in your spouse's ear, blowing lightly on the skin and nibbling the ears.

Some couples might enjoy eating different foods or chocolate from each other's bodies. A few suggestions include strawberries and cream, chocolates and some people recommend things like honey or ice. But use whatever tickles your taste buds!

The setting. The setting you create may cause you to feel turned-on and sexually excited. Experiment by creating a Western setting and wearing cowboy and cowgirl outfits while having sex. You may want to try a Hawaiian setting with flowers and swimming costumes and massage oil. Being creative with the setting and your clothing may create an atmosphere that puts both you and your spouse in the right mood for fabulous sex.

Other turn-ons. Removal of body hair may be very attractive to some people; it adds to the body feeling touch and caress. Wives can shave under their armpits, around the nipples, their legs, or their pubic hair into shapes or all off. Husbands, you can either trim hair on all parts of your body or shave it off. Some wives prefer a bit of facial hair on their husbands but discuss this between you. Some couples may find cleanly shaved bodies or body parts exciting while other prefer the natural look. This may also be culturally related so open communication is once again the answer.

Complete honesty can be a wonderful sexual turn-on, trusting your spouse with very personal information about yourself. This also indicates a deeper level in your relationship because you are trusting your spouse with very intimate details.

Determining what turns your spouse on sexually is a matter of communicating with them about what you like and dislike. In this way you do not only get to know each other more intimately, but you also give your spouse the opportunity to sexually turn you on.

Remember, it is not an impossible task to know what turns you on and what turns you off. Your spouse is not a mind reader and you should openly tell your partner what you like and what you dislike. Do not be shy! Be courageous and allow your spouse to spoil you by doing exactly what you enjoy.

8.3 Romance

Romance is what sets the mood for sex, the catalyst for sexual excitement resulting in awesome sexual intercourse and fulfilment.

Love letters are a great way of exciting your spouse. Telling your spouse in writing how incredibly sexy he or she is and exactly how much you would like to have sex with them and the way you want to can be incredibly sexually inviting. Romantic love letters describe the moment within a moment. Here is an example of a love letter a wife wrote to her husband:

'My love, my strong man, my incredibly wonderful husband! Could you be anymore handsome? Passion glows in my face when I think about your clear eyes, incredible manly smile, your focussed attention

on me. My breasts and nipples turn firm a tension, alive. Do you see my femininity inviting your every intention? I long for your rough, big hands on my body and your warm breath in my neck. I feel faint when you look at me as if you want to consume me for yourself and make us one. I love you so much. Our Creator has blessed me with you, a man like no other. I shall be faithful to death. I will be forever grateful to Him. I cannot wait for our next moment of romance and I will endeavour to entice you so you will not be able to wait for our passionate encounter. I love you.'

If you would like a burning hot romantic letter, write about the last time you made love to your spouse and enjoyed it tremendously. Here is an example of a letter a husband wrote to his wife:

'My sweet love, I was trying to stay focussed today, but was passionately distracted by my thoughts of your lovely body last night, hearing your heavy breathing indicating how much you wanted me as I stroked your thighs. You were tilting your head back, opening your mouth and moving your body rhythmically; do you ever realise how much I love you? The ringing of the phone now at work made me put down my pen and turn back to reality, but to no avail, when I answered and heard your gentle voice on the other side, whispering to my heart. I am burning with passion, like a wild stallion driven to run and catch up to you, let us explore, let us love until sunrise. I want to hold you again, disclosing your intimate secrets only to myself when you turn uncontrollably wild; would you let me? I want to feel your gentle touch, your sweet caresses, smell your perfume, and see your warm skin tingle; you are mine. I love you.'

Romance is the moment within the moment, which can happen spontaneously or be created, depending on the preferences of the couple. A romantic moment or evening is an event where more time is spent to create it, more creative power invested into it so more than one or all of the senses are actively taking in information. Sensing so much information can feel like the time is slowing down and the moment is coming to a perfect stop to be perfectly absorbed.

Different venues can be romantic to different individuals. This is what makes a marriage so wonderfully special, exploring the different romantic venues together. Your spouse might like nature and you might like the comfort of service delivery in a hotel. It would be wise to accommodate both yourself and your spouse or take turns when choosing venues.

Moving your bodies together, dancing, looking at each other and being intimate can be incredibly romantic. All the senses and parts of the bodies touch while dancing, causing tremendous sexual sensations when meant for this purpose. Here we are not referring to ballroom dancing, but private, romantic, sexually stimulating dancing between a husband and wife.

Being alone with your spouse without the children or family and friends around can be romantic. Just sensing each other and being aware of each other only can cause a romantic atmosphere.

Romance can be what you choose it to be, causing you and your spouse to spend a great night together enjoying each other's company.

Your romantic engagement does not have to end in sexual intercourse. Romance is a building tool in your relationship. It is founded in trust. You and your spouse need to be able to trust each other first and foremost to be able to be courageous and spontaneous. It is important to be mature, to be the adult you are. You can be spontaneous, but try never to be insensitive or childish as this will only diminish your romantic relationship.

Some couples take a day off from work and spend time together, just being alone and naked at home. When doing so you do not have to engage sexually, but if you do, it could be the ultimate fulfilment. Just being different together builds trust and feelings of romance. Trusting your secrets to each other will cause you both to be more romantic.

Visualise putting a crown on your spouse's head, honouring your spouse once again the way God wants you to. Laying your life down for the one you love as one, asking the Lord to help you to keep this in place is indeed romantic, because there is trust and honour involved. Both spouses can do this for each other in prayer.

Get your thinking juices flowing and create your own romantic ideas to put passion power back into your marriage and put joy into your romance.

8.4 Cleanliness

Cleanliness is founded in simple choice and action while being a three-fold process, based on the three dimensions the Bible mentions when talking about the spirit, soul and body.[53]

The spirit is clean when you are born again and serve God through loving your spouse. This love may be tamed or untamed, but this is unconditional love. Keeping your spirit clean is based on living a life of purity and holiness. Forgiveness is the first step towards cleanliness; living a life of forgiveness and holding nothing against any other person. Honesty in everything, even when it is really difficult, is the second step towards a life of cleanliness. Sin causes the spirit to become unclean and sin is not only about the so-called 'big sins' like adultery, but also missing the mark, in other words, not doing exactly what you know God expects of you. You cannot become sinless all of a sudden; first admit your sin and realise we are sinful people, then repent and move on.

The soul consists of the will, the emotions and the thoughts, and is clean when it is humbly submitted to the will of God. When you have thoughts or plans outside the will of God, you need to take them captive while submitting them to the Lord. Let your mind be pleasing to God in everything. This means forsaking your own will for the will of God. Doing His will in your life regardless of what your thoughts and emotions tell you. His will for your life is to love Him above all else and then to love your spouse unconditionally[54]. Your soul becomes unclean when you think, feel or do anything contrary to the will of God, thus rejecting the guidance of the Holy Spirit.

The body can be kept clean by living a healthy life and through taking care of it by washing regularly and dressing appropriately. Exercise regularly. Cleaning your body, making yourself look and smell good does not only impress your spouse, but it also portrays you as a representative of the Most High God on earth, and you thus treat yourself accordingly. The body gets unclean by living a promiscuous life, eating and drinking unhealthily and doing no exercise.

8.5 Summary

Invest time and optimism in your sex life and you will enjoy the benefits for years to come. Your creativity can make it grow into something really special and beautiful. Give yourself the freedom to invest in your sex life and free the hidden spontaneity in both you and your spouse. Be courageous!

Sex is a wonderful gift that God gave humans to enjoy within the boundaries of marriage, but enjoying sex is every married individual's responsibility. You should take up this responsibility and clearly determine what you like and what you dislike. Then you should take it a step further and clearly and openly communicate with your spouse about your likes and dislikes. By doing this you are setting the stage for your spouse to help you become sexually fulfilled by doing exactly what you like and long for.

Your responsibility for a great sex life starts with romance that has nothing to do with direct sexual intercourse. Romantic moments may be created to create a mood for sex, but romance should be a way of life. Be romantic towards your spouse throughout the day in the way you relate, communicate and behave towards each other. Your love should naturally flow into romance, constant touch and closeness between you. Physical, emotional and spiritual intimacy will naturally flow over into a sexually fulfilled marriage.

Cleanliness costs nothing, but it is your responsibility to keep yourself clean in spirit, soul and body in order to be the best possible spouse you are able to be.

Take the responsibility then to share your sexual turn-ons and turn-offs with your spouse and actively pursue the fulfilment of your spouse's turn-ons while avoiding the turn-offs.

Are you excited about embarking on a whole new chapter of an honest, fulfilling and spontaneous sexual adventure with your spouse?

CHAPTER 9

Sexual activities and positions

9.1 Desire

Desire is sacred and therefore we believe it is one of God's secrets meant to be shared only in a marriage. If you are married, desiring someone other than your spouse is called temptation, the first step to sin.

However, spiritual desire happens when you draw closer to God by among other things, embracing the masculinity or femininity that He bestowed on you. As a man, you have strength a woman could never have, you have a penis and sperm a woman will never have and you are the leader of your home. As a woman, you have beauty beyond measure which God has bestowed upon you just because you are a woman, you are protected by your husband and the kingdom of God, you produce milk through your beautiful breasts, and are able to carry God-given life in your body. These liberating thoughts are the first steps towards desire and to creating a platform for sexual desire.

As a wife towards your husband or as a husband towards your wife, living in truth (transparency) towards one another, being mature and naked close together equals emotional desire.

A healthy emotional desire shows spouses what to do when they are together without having to say everything in words. For instance, when you have an electrifying feeling flowing through your breasts and your husband picks up on this and rubs them while, for instance, kissing you, or your wife cuddles straight into your arms while you are thinking about it so you can hold her beautiful body against you. These are breathless moments.

And yes, it is terrible when your emotional desire plunges when you and your spouse do not meet each other at the same point of sexual desire, causing frustration. A wise couple meets honestly at that point by applying unconditional love and giving each other the glory to create a healthy balance. In practice, do what your spouse wants before you make them do what you want. This leads us to discuss emotional maturity in your relationship.

Maturity is very important but so is grace and mercy for the sake of peace. Let's give each other the grace to mature with time, like a good year in wine. You will be amazed by the wonderful person God created for you to marry when they have grown to emotional maturity You will be delighted by the fruits you have been waiting to pick. Being gracefully patient will benefit your investment in your future together and your emotional desire towards each other will be kept intact. When your emotional desire is temporarily strained, it is wise to look at your spouse through God's eyes for every good attribute. Meditate on those good qualities together with the Holy Spirit and consciously stay away from thoughts that will cause bad habits.

Emotional desire takes action when your emotions, thoughts and will become one with God and your spouse. You both want to reach out to each other in a very private manner, being yourself in complete honesty. How much is there to hide in total nakedness, openness and oneness? How much do you want to express your desires to your spouse and how much do you want your spouse to express their desires to you? Expressing your sexual emotions, expressing desirable thoughts and seeing how your spouse welcomes your expressions will be immense turn-ons.

Physical desire is when your body and actions speak out loud; the eyes say 'I want to see you', the mouth says 'I want to taste you', the nose says 'I want to smell you', the heart says 'I want you', your mind desires every part of your spouse as much as your heart does, your genitals respond to wanting your spouse and wanting to give yourself to your spouse! This incredible feeling merges together with romance and foreplay. When physical desire is in full swing, the next step is intercourse.

Unconditional desire in a woman for her husband only comes into the full when she is married to him. Sleeping together before you are married might bring some pleasure through sin, but it will not set the woman free from feeling insecure.

How do we stimulate desire, and is it possible? Yes! Good and positive thoughts and actions definitely stimulate desire. Desire is not predictable. This is why people can fall in love with each other over and over within the marriage. It is possible, wonderful and very exciting; however, remember unconditional love is the glue in your marriage.

You might be walking down the aisles of a grocery store and find your spouse's loving eyes desiring you. You might not even know what it is that makes you desirable to your spouse. You might be balancing the books and suddenly you find her staring at you with those 'come-to-bed eyes', and you are blown out of the water because you forgot to buy her flowers but she wants you NOW!

You might be changing the oil of the car and you see her eyes running you over through the opening between the bonnet and the car. It will be a moment in which you'll know she wants to be intimate with you. The secret to this wonderful gift God gave your marriage is to accumulate these wonderful, desirous moments between you and your wife. When the pastor of your church speaks about investing in your marriage or filling the love cup, these are the moments to which they are usually referring.

When you build on the desire between you and your spouse, foreplay might become a shorter venture, so make sure to keep desire alive.

It is a great idea to ask your spouse what it is they desire about you, and it is just as appealing to drop a hint on what you desire; it could even open a discussion leading to a very intimate moment between you before sexual intercourse.

The Bible speaks about desire and one full book was dedicated to it. Take a look at the *Songs of Solomon* written by King Solomon, which is packed with sexual desire, romance, love and passion. When you apply those words to your spouse, you will be able to feel the desire described there. One example is Song of Songs 1:1: 'Let him kiss me with the kisses of his mouth – for your love is more delightful than wine. Pleasing is the fragrance of your perfumes; your name is like perfume poured out. No wonder the maidens love you!' We can translate this to mean: 'Kiss me passionately – your love is faithful and safe to me. Pleasing is the fragrance of your aftershave; big businessmen refer to you with respect. No wonder all the ladies admire you!' So now you can be creative and make your own desirable thoughts about your spouse.

Proverbs 19:22 teaches, 'what is desired in a man is kindness, and a poor man is better than a liar.[55]' The Bible says it out straight: when you are kind to your wife, you are expressing your desire. When your spouse reacts to this, her response will be desire in return. The Bible says in the manner in which you give you will receive, so how about exploring in full your kindness towards your wife?

So what is the difference between lust and desire? It is a very fine distinct line. Lust happens when a person is uncontrollably sexually self-indulgent. The person is driven by a force or feeling of inadequacy and therefore seeks sexual empowerment over another. Lust seeks to manipulate or control and the end result is condemnation, guilt and again, inadequacy, emptiness or loneliness. This incredibly inadequate feeling can be dealt with in prayer, deep inner healing and deliverance through your church.

Lust steals from people, it promises fulfilment, but in the end gives endless emptiness. You might even believe you are pleasing someone by sexually enticing them or having hard sex with them, where in fact it might be painful or very uncomfortable and humiliating. When a lustful person is apprehended, the situation will most likely turn into a fight or guilt or condemnation, maybe even rejection or in some really bad cases, violence.

Thoughts that lust empowers are thoughts like, 'you can please me', 'I will make you do this or that', 'you cannot live without me', 'I will make you scream', and 'you will beg'. Lust seeks to destroy, so it feeds on fear and timidity.

Desire is good and acceptable. Desire between spouses is a humble, searching energy from one spouse to the other. The desire energy draws spouses near to each other and encouragingly empowers them to interact with the other's expression of sexual intimacy needs with a goal of pre-sexual pleasure. What does this mean? This means that when the man expresses kindness in the form of desire to his wife, he empowers her or energises her to react to his signal of sexual intimacy. When she reacts to his signal by, for instance, moving her body in a sexy manner or smiling, she again empowers or energises his desire for her.

This is what memories between spouses are made with. How can you ever forget the first time your husband opened the door for you, or carried you across the threshold? How can you ever forget how your wife tossed her hair over her shoulder and smiled at you when you opened the door for her? This is the glue between you and your spouse; it keeps you warm at night and cosy in the winter, hot and perky in the summer and smiling most of the time.

You can prepare yourself to be desired by your spouse. A man can make a note to be kind to his wife, unconditionally. It will be challenging at times, but hey, you can do it! A wife can focus on engaging with the kindness of her husband through being the sensual lady she is. While with the children, you will be in mother-mode, while being playful or teasing, you might be in child-mode, but being in adult-mode is where you want to fully experience the fullness of God's intention in the bedroom.

Sometimes we can be really spiteful towards our spouse by being deliberately lazy. We all get to that point sometimes! Move your intentions away from the devil and your positive energy towards your spouse by being really good. For a change we can work with God to make our sexual experience glow and glowing; it will, when desire is healthy.

Thoughts communicated with the Lord of desire energises, for instance, 'Lord, You created him handsomely or 'Lord, You made her so beautiful' and with that might come a feeling of intense thankfulness towards God for being able to engage sexually with your spouse. Or 'how can I please you more?', 'I want to be with you', 'I need you with me', 'let's be together', 'let me hold you close to my heart', 'I love you so much' etc.

Feeling desire means looking for opportunities and building the results into great memories, and practise, practise, practise. To consciously build on the good points in your sexual relationship will make it strong, and to consciously strengthen the weak points will bring a great selection of choices of all the good and strong points. This should not be a secret as God wants you to enjoy yourself.

Use your sexual journal to write down all the ideas you would like to remember.

9.2 Foreplay

Sex is a gift from God for couples to enjoy each other within the boundaries of marriage. God created sex so involve Him through the guidance of the Holy Spirit in your sex life and move towards sexual fulfilment. Some wonderful biblical pointers on foreplay, as well as valuable guiding principles for your love making, are found in the Song of Solomon. Song of Solomon 1:1-17 and 2:1-17 are excellent examples of this.

God created the sexual act and intended for it to work under the guidance of the Holy Spirit; it is therefore not difficult to realise why non-believers do not find true sexual fulfilment and satisfaction. True sexual fulfilment can only be experienced when the Creator of sex is involved in the act and his ways are followed. Invite the Holy Spirit into your bedroom the next time you and your spouse engage in sexual intercourse. Ask Him what to do next and listen; you will experience his guidance and 'inside information' in taking your sex life to a whole new level.

Foreplay involves studying and exploring every part of your spouse's body. Spend time just being together, touching each other, while taking special notice of what sexually excites your spouse and remembering it for future use. Spend time giving pleasure without expecting anything in return. The focus should be on your spouse and the way he or she responds to your interaction.

Look at your spouse; truly look at each part of his or her body. Hold your spouse while touching and admiring, in this way showing your love. Touch your spouse's hand, gently squeeze it and continue foreplay by just feeling the softness of her skin or the firmness of his muscles under your hands.

It sounds like a first date, but it really is not. Every woman wants to feel admired for her beauty and the beauty inside her. She wants to know when you think she is kind-hearted, loving, helpful, caring, giving and gentle, because these things matter to her on a daily basis. A husband being close to you because he admires you is more noticeable than when his words are not carried over into actions. Find those special points of admiration in your wife and work on yourself to keep on admiring her for how God created her beauty.

Every man wants to feel competent and wanted and therefore every wife should never reject her husband or make him feel inferior. Always make him feel respected and good about himself. Support him, love him and just be a loving wife to him, while admiring him for being a man of God and a great lover trying to please you and sexually satisfy you.

Love is not a feeling. Love is a decision you should make on a daily basis and when you consciously behave lovingly towards your spouse, your feelings will align with your decision. You are building the success of tomorrow, today.

Loving your spouse should be shown in your words, deeds and behaviour. Believe in love. Use your imagination on how you would like to explore your wife's beauty and fine contours, or your husband's firm and strong body during foreplay. Foreplay can be lots of fun and is about being close to each other, involving the skin as much as possible and making your spouse feel desired and close to you.

A husband, while waiting for his wife to return home from work, ran a hot bath for her and filled it with rose petals. He took care of dinner, thus removing any concerns she might have had, and put on soft background music. When she came home, he called her to the bedroom, undressed her slowly while kissing her, picked her up and put her into the bathtub. He then began to wash every part of her body, exploring her beauty, gently massaging her scalp, causing her to relax and forget about all the day's stresses. After washing her, he offered his hand and helped her out of the bath. He gently dried her, kissing the parts of her body he found inviting, then proceeded by lying her down on their bed. He took body lotion and slowly massaged it into her feet, legs and inner thighs, her buttocks, tummy, breasts, arms and neck, while kissing her all over her body. This considerate form of foreplay ended with the two of them relaxing in each other's arms after having fulfilling sex.

A few things you may use to create a romantic atmosphere leading to excellent foreplay include a feather for gentle stroking, whispering, a love letter, singing, intimate kissing, massaging, soft background music, candles, a bath filled with aromatic water, a soft scent to spray in the air, romantic soft lighting and expectant spontaneity.

During foreplay your spouse might reach a sexual climax and orgasm even without intending to, but do not be angry or disappointed; the same might happen to you, so be humble and enjoy it with your spouse. Let your spouse enjoy the experience and thereafter your partner should help you reach orgasm as well. If you are the wife who reached orgasm during foreplay, be glad and continue enjoying the sexual experience as you may reach another orgasm, or more. If you are the husband who reached orgasm during foreplay and ejaculated, continue to sexually please your wife and help her reach orgasm either through manual stimulation, oral sex or by using a sex toy. Reaching orgasm during foreplay should never be the end of your sexual time together; just continue intercourse.

Massage is a great method of foreplay; it increases touch while reducing stress. To massage the scalp, let your spouse lie down, then firmly but gently use your fingers to stroke and play with their hair, brushing your fingers through it. Let the tips of your fingers firmly massage the scalp, moving the skin in small, circular movements, then take the hair between your fingers and make your hands into fists so the hair gently pulls the skin on their scalp. Let go and take new bunches of hair, pulling the skin on the scalp gently, then massaging with your fingertips again. Cover the whole head. You can gently rub and pull the ears to enhance the blood flow and create a relaxed feeling.

To massage the body, make use of massage oil or body lotion; pour some into your hands and rub the hands together over the part which is going to be massaged, so the oil drips on the skin and warms between your hands. Gently but firmly rub the skin, moving your hands to create a sensation of touch and calmness. Massage around bone to relax the muscle around it. Avoid putting pressure on the bone structure as this may be uncomfortable. Where the body has more skin and fat, deeper massaging can be applied, but always be gently firm. Because this is a foreplay massage, you can massage the genitals and breasts. What can also be very arousing is to massage your spouse's body without any oil or body lotion, concentrating on skin against skin to heighten the feeling of closeness and intimacy.

Do not rely on movies to do your foreplay for you. Pornography will deceive you into thinking that everyone should look perfect and that sex can continue for hours and hours without ever having to stop. It misrepresents sex and will only cause you to compare yourself to what they portray to be true. The adult entertainment industry sends a false message to the world with the sex scenes it portrays on television or in movies. A husband or wife watching a movie filled with those perceptions may be disappointed in reality. The problem is not with the wife or the husband; the problem is with unrealistic expectations.

A husband and wife had some fun one evening when she decided to act like a movie star. They began making love and she was throwing her hair around and moaning while jumping up and down, like she'd seen in the movies. She thought he would have the most fun ever and would ask for it again and again, but instead he giggled uncontrollably, and it was that end of the movie performance!

On a different note, molestation rates may be worse or just reported more effectively these days, so keep in mind that your spouse might knowingly or unknowingly be part of those statistics in the form of a victim. Have compassion towards each other and be willing to seek help should a sexual problem exist and persist. It is not a sign of weakness to ask a professional person for help, but rather a sure indication of your willingness to deal with the problem in order to overcome it. When you reach out and seek help, you are being humble because you are not only doing it for yourself; you are doing it for those who love you. When seeking professional help, seek a properly qualified and experienced therapist who makes use of a Christian value system.

Optimistic body language is a great trigger for sexual foreplay. Being joyful and excited about the moment may bring a whole new flavour to the bedroom.

For the marriage and sexual relationship to stay strong, you need to spend time with your spouse; spiritually, emotionally and physically. The wife was created as the husband's help meet.[56] Spending time with your spouse, helping with whatever activity, will bond the two of you which will make it easier to engage sexually. Remember, as the wife you are supposed to be a helper; nothing more and nothing less. You are not an advisor, counsellor, manager, slave or money saver, but helper when he asks for help or even when he does not. Determine the way you want to help in line with your responsibility towards God. You are responsible for your growth in faith just as he is responsible for his own personal growth in faith.

Being sexy even while being holy is a very attractive quality in a spouse. You do not have to *make* yourself sexy, you just need to believe you are wonderfully made by God and this inner knowing will result in you being attractive and sexy. Get to know yourself and tell your spouse what you like and how to eagerly respond. Take responsibility for your own sexual fulfilment and share it with your spouse. Never blame your spouse for not knowing what you want if you do not want to communicate openly and share the information with him or her.

9.2.1 Holding hands

Regardless of how long you have been married, holding hands is always a great way to get close to your spouse. It helps you to become aware of your spouse's presence and love by just being together. Holding hands is not only for friends, it is also a building tool for married couples.

Holding hands can be very special. Next time you sit with your spouse, slide your hand into theirs, hold it a while and while looking at your spouse, gently squeeze until your palms touch and hold it there for a moment while you look away, then just hold their hand. Do not let go, keep your hands interlinked. Even while making love, this is a great way of being intimate. While having sex in the missionary position (see page xx) and you are on top, put both your interlinked hands into your spouse's hands and just hold them firmly while sexually engaging. The intimacy might be electrifying.

Another way is to let the fingertips and the palms touch while looking at each other. This is also a great intimacy builder.

9.2.2 French kissing

French kissing is one of the most passionate, loving ways to engage in as foreplay, together with hugging and touching. The combination needs practise because you need to go with the flow of the increased sexual excitement. Pressing too hard or stroking too softly with your hands and arms while kissing might be a turn-off, so practise, practise, practise. Always remember that there is no right or wrong way of French kissing.

French kissing is when you and your spouse kiss by using your tongues. In a very relaxed sexually private atmosphere, you can look into each other's eyes or at your spouse's mouth, slowly move closer while tilting your head slightly to the side and slightly opening your mouth, while breathing in. At this point you can close your eyes or keep them open; it's your choice.

Feel your spouse's mouth with your lips while opening your mouth a little more. Feel your spouse's breathing, the warmth of their mouth and the wetness of their tongue as you both touch each other with your tongues. Do not hold your tongue still at any time and do not move it rhythmically in the same direction; be creative. Move your tongue in different positions, keeping it to the front part of your spouse's mouth, maybe slightly deeper to the middle and as passion increases, you might kiss deeply. Occasionally lick your spouse's lips while sucking slightly either their tongue or the lips. You can breathe in through your mouth and breath out through your nose. Be creative and become a great kisser.

This is such a wonderful way to engage in becoming one with your spouse. The intimacy-building factor of this motion is almost indescribable. When fantasising about the night before, French kissing is almost always part of the sexual memory.

It causes a wonderful sensation to change the direction of your head, tilting and moving it to the other side and back again while passionately kissing. At the same time use your hands and arms to hold, rub or squeeze different parts of your spouse's body to create sexual tension.

Sometimes when a spouse becomes really turned-on, they relax the focus of kissing. Kissing too hard is only nice when the person being kissed also likes it. Check with your spouse before kissing them with your tongue right to the back of their mouth, licking their teeth or between the teeth and lips or touching teeth, or biting their tongue (even lovingly, some people might not like it).

Try to end your French kiss with a soft kiss on the lips to indicate to your spouse you will be ending the kiss. This is not compulsory, but it is good manners since no-one wants to be left with an unmet expectation. Without breaking the atmosphere of sexual expectation, you may continue by kissing the rest of the body.

If you are really insecure about your kissing skills, ask for your spouse's honest feedback or better still practise, practise and practise. Homework never sounded so good, especially when you are advised to practise kissing until you feel you are good at it! You were not born knowing how to kiss, although it is quite a natural manner of loving, and it is perfectly normal to feel a little insecure about it. This insecurity can be overcome with practise.

Some couples might prefer engaging in manual sex while French kissing. This is a naturally wonderful progression of French kissing, preparing the genitals of both spouses for sexual intercourse.

Mutual masturbation is a wonderful way to get you to be equally sexually excited.

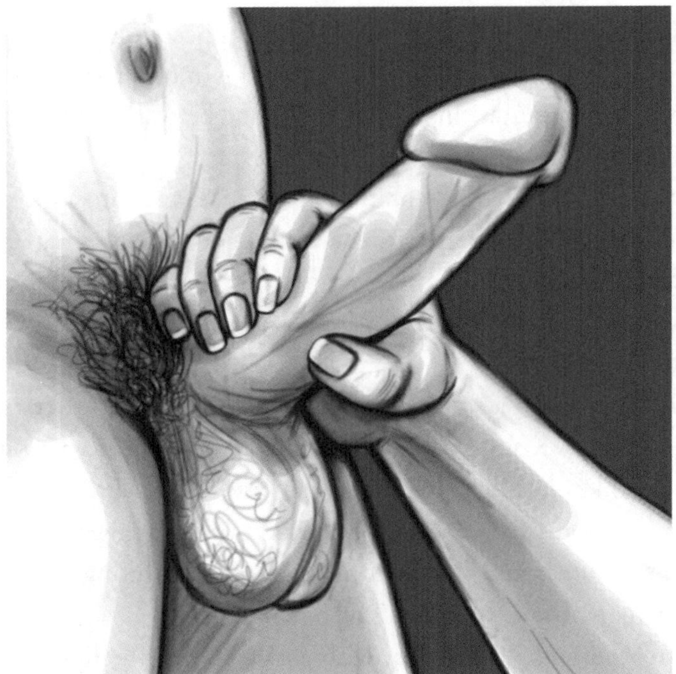

How do you masturbate the penis? Gently stroke the body to indicate your movement towards the penis's shaft. Gently rub over the whole area of the penis and scrotum, but do not squeeze the scrotum. Glide your one hand over the penis shaft as shown in the diagram and put your other hand just underneath the scrotum, applying firm pressure. Gently start from the base of the penis and pull to the end of the penis, slightly let go and return to the base and repeat. The penis will rapidly enlarge as this procedure is continued. When the penis is erect, the pace and pressure can be readjusted. This is just a basic suggestion and can be varied with your husband's choice or your initiative.

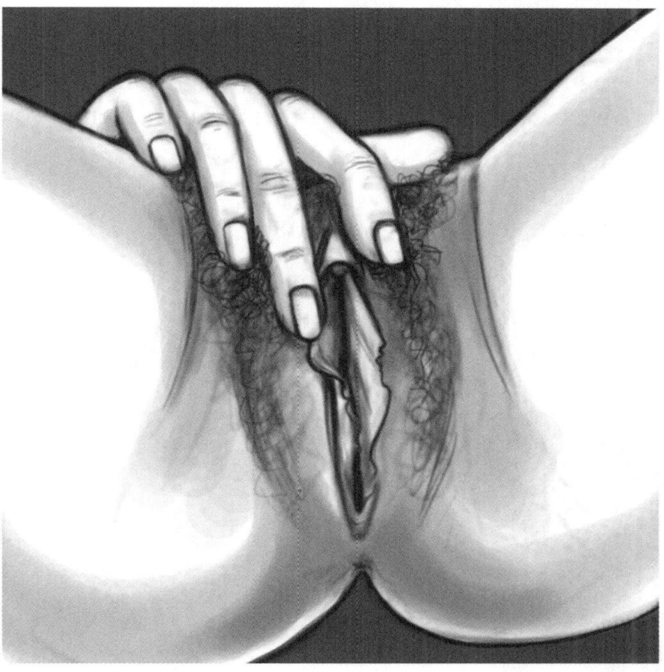

How do you masturbate the clitoris and vagina? Allow enough time not to rush this to ensure that your spouse is relaxed. Again, this is a basic suggestion; you and your spouse may develop your own manner of masturbating the clitoris and vagina. After stimulating the vulva by gently rubbing and stroking with or without lubrication over the area of the labia, gently take the clitoris between your index finger and thumb. Make circular movements clockwise and anti-clockwise until the clitoris becomes erect and continue until your wife reaches orgasm;

climaxing may occur several times. To bring deeper emotion between you, apply the palm of your hand over the pubic bone, gently but firmly pushing upwards over the clitoris area, thus massaging the vulva upwards while you both breathe in deeply, resulting into a powerful emotional state of intimacy. Continue breathing deeply while looking into your spouse's eyes.

Apply your forefinger and middle finger to the vagina and penetrate while stimulating the walls of the vagina. Right behind the clitoris is a soft, spongy tissue, covering the wall of the vagina; this is the G-spot. Communicate with your spouse about finding a wonderful way to stimulate the G-spot with either firm movements or a 'come-here' finger motion, palm upwards.

9.3 Different sexual positions

There are numerous sexual positions and the best way of knowing what works for you and what doesn't is to try them out; experiment with various sexual positions. Never be afraid to try new things. You may like

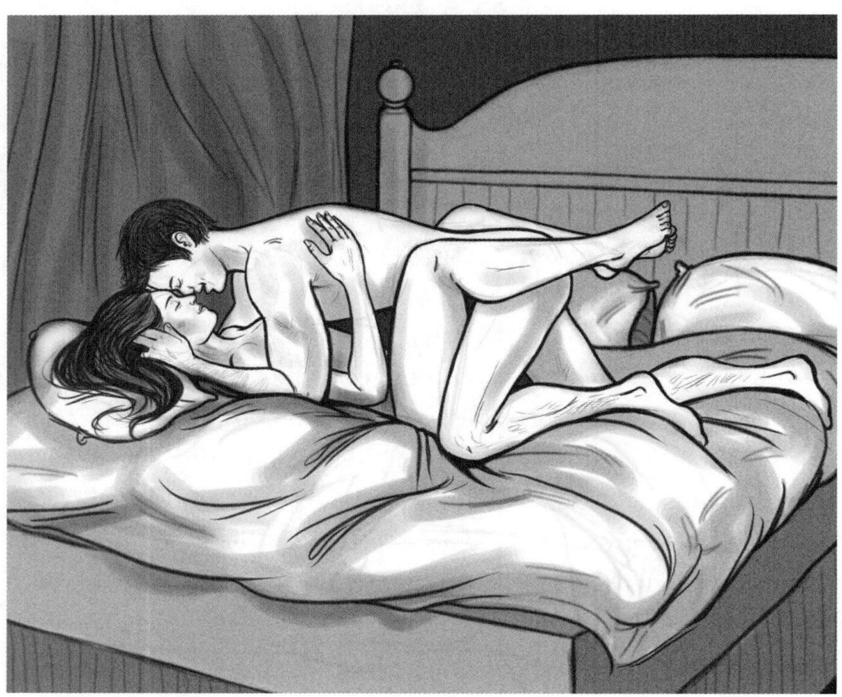

certain positions and use them more often or you may not like certain positions and never use them again, or only use them occasionally if your spouse enjoys them. Always remember that sex does not have to become boring and predictable; use different positions to spice up your sex life.

9.3.1 The missionary position

The missionary position is the most familiar and probably the best position with which to start off where the husband lies on top of his wife. Occasionally change the venue for sex from the bed to other places in the house and in this way the same position may bring about more excitement due to a change in scenery. When the husband has a secure place to put his feet against, like a wall, a steady couch or the edge of the bed, it might help with penetration, giving it a whole different feel.

Here is a basic description and some pointers on making love in the missionary position; every person will have their own style, but this is just a basic template from which you can start.

After foreplay, being nicely lubricated, open the labia areas on both sides of the vagina before inserting the penis into the vagina as an alternative to just penetrating. Glide the penis in firm and fast instead of the normal careful penetration, just for the purpose of increased sensation. Husbands may firmly push their pubic area against their wives' vulva by using their buttocks and not only their back, as if trying to move her upwards. Keep it there for a few seconds and then pull back to the opening of the vagina and push back inside. You may then find a pace that is comfortable for you both to begin thrusting.

You may want to stimulate the whole vulval area with the beginning of your shaft as you push in and pull out every time. Nerve endings on the whole vulval area are susceptible to sensation, not just inside the vagina. Pushing upwards will involve the clitoris more directly, making it a more complete arousal. It is very important for the husband to keep up the pace (not necessarily move faster) until the wife reaches orgasm and for a little while thereafter. You may either reach your climax together, but whatever you decide is your choice.

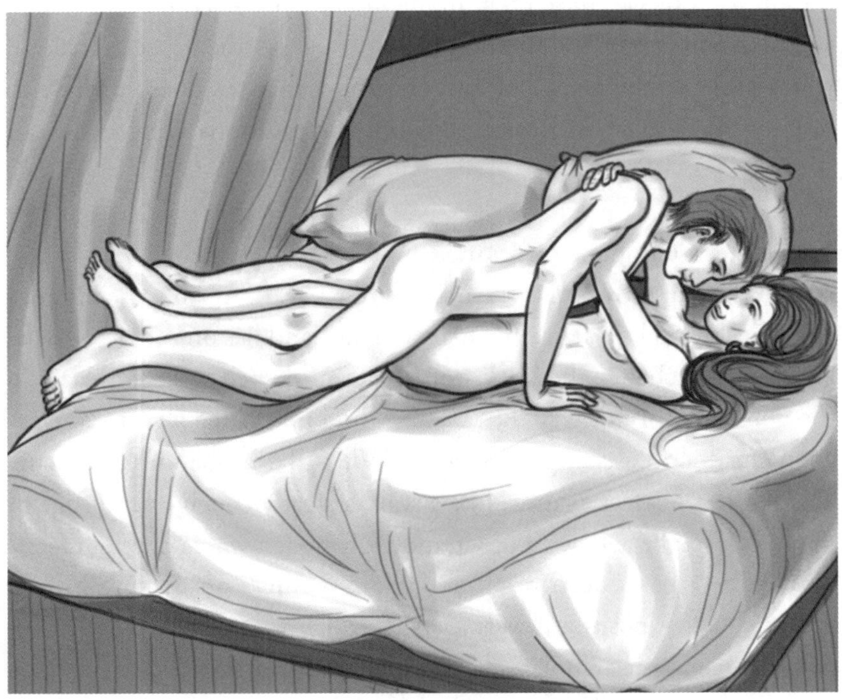

When you have both reached orgasm, you may slow the rhythm down, just kissing and holding each other, keeping emotional contact and just intimately relaxing in your spouse's arms. Some couples like talking afterwards, some do not; it is up to you and your spouse what you would like to do, but whatever you decide, keep close contact during this time. The plateau stage after orgasm is just as important as intercourse itself to increase intimacy between you.

The wife may want to contract the vagina while her husband pulls his penis out and relax the muscles while he penetrates again.

The wife may actually exercise these muscles by practising when she goes to urinate; practise by doing the following: urinate, hold back the urine for two seconds and then urinate again and once again hold back for two seconds, and so forth until urination is completed. This will cause her to have more control over the muscles, putting her in more control of regulating her orgasms during sexual intercourse.

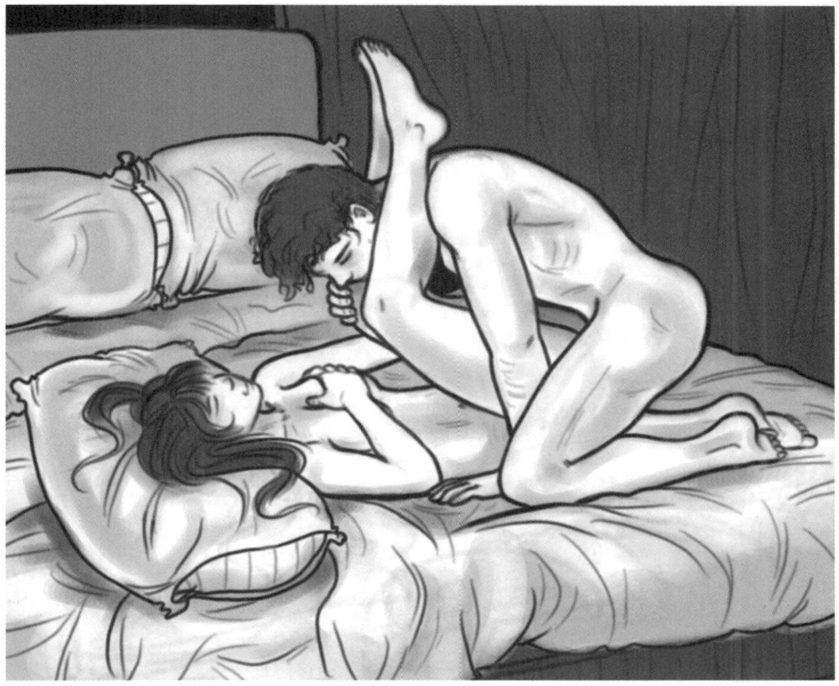

A variation to the missionary position is for the wife to open her legs and when the husband penetrates her, to actually close her legs and move them in underneath her husband's body. This position intensifies the pressure inside the vagina.

Another variation of the missionary position is when the wife straightens her legs against her husband's chest with her feet next to his head. When doing this the husband is actually standing on his knees. When placing his knees on both sides of his wife's buttocks, the husband is actually in a good position to control and delay ejaculation, giving his wife more time to reach orgasm and maybe to experience multiple orgasms.

The relaxed position is partially a variation of the missionary position. It is absolutely wonderful for overweight spouses as penetration is fulfilling. A pregnant wife should also be comfortable in this position. The wife simply lies with her two legs in between her husband's legs, enabling them to enjoy sexual intercourse.

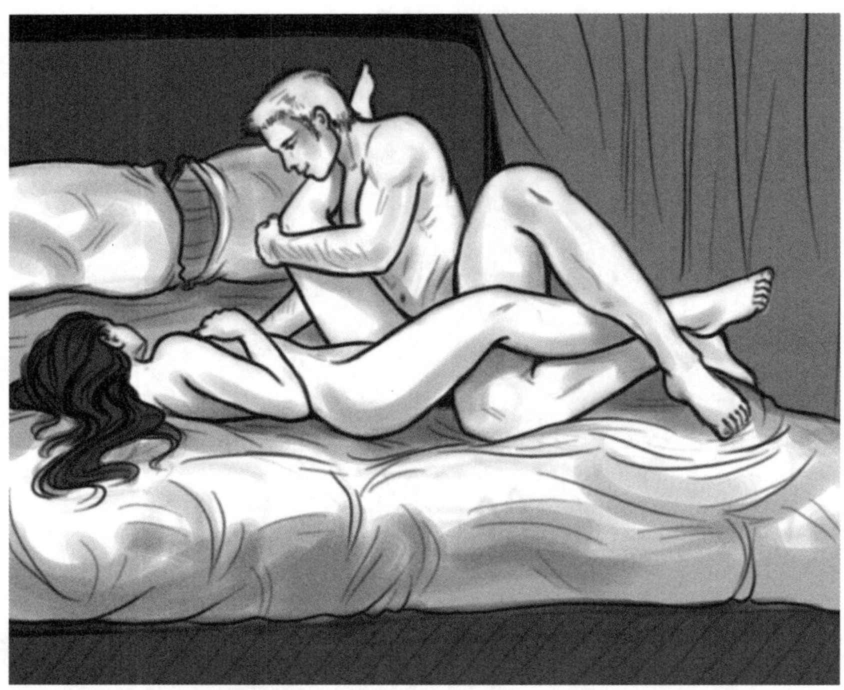

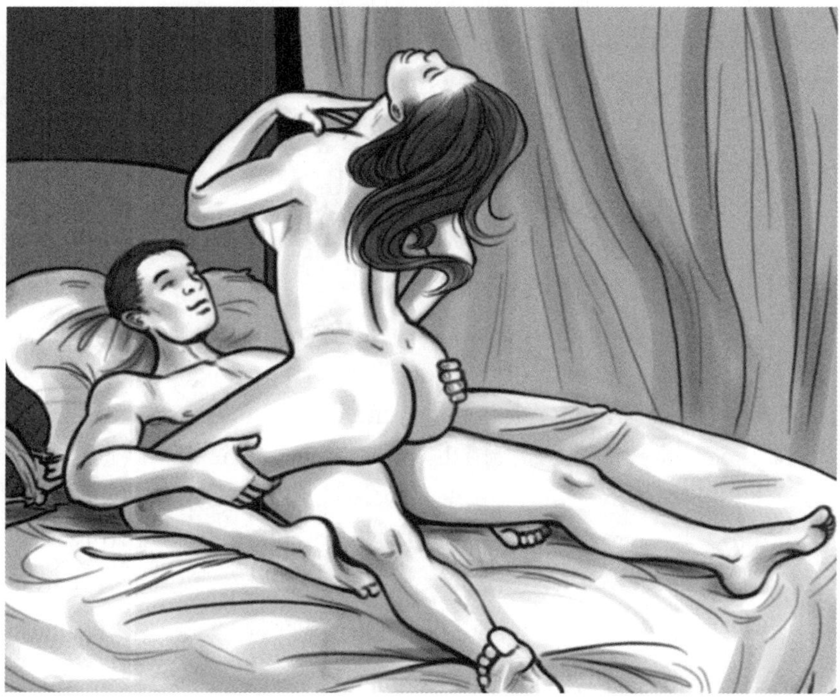

9.3.2 Wife-on-top position

The wife-on-top position is an excellent position when the woman wants to take a more active and dominating role in the sex act. It is a huge turn-on for most men and a great position when the husband is tired or lacks energy. The husband will find this position highly arousing since he will have his hands free to touch his wife, look at her and enjoy the sexual experience while his wife is in control.

This position will allow the wife to have control over the depth, motion and frequency of penetration. This is a great position for a pregnant wife. The wife will be able to move around as she pleases and be in total control of her orgasm. The husband's hands are free and he may touch her breasts, hold her sides, hold her buttocks or even play with her clitoris during sexual intercourse. For an intimate touch, he may hold her face in his hands.

The wife holds her legs straight, but as a variation she may bend them and actually sit on her knees, giving her even more control over her own body movements.

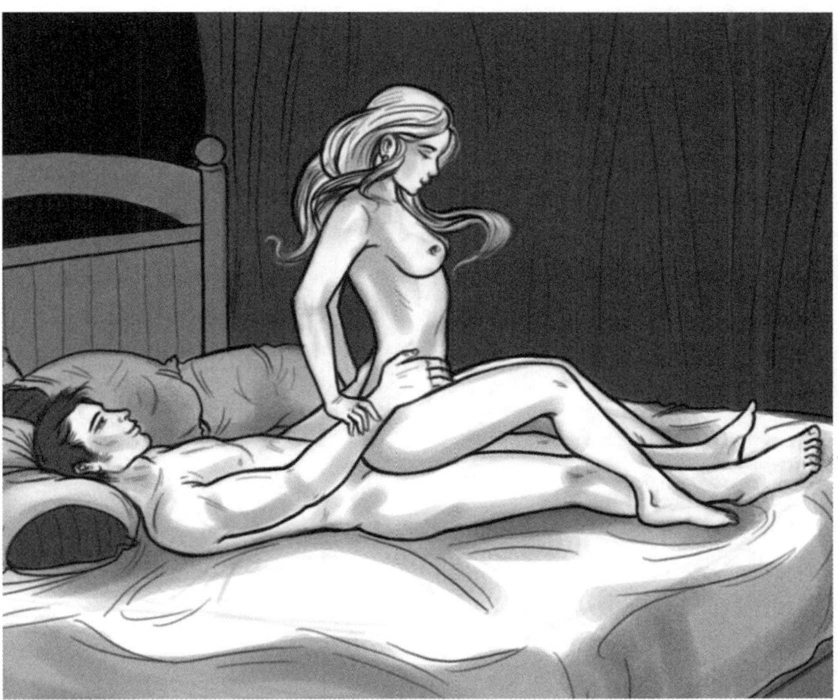

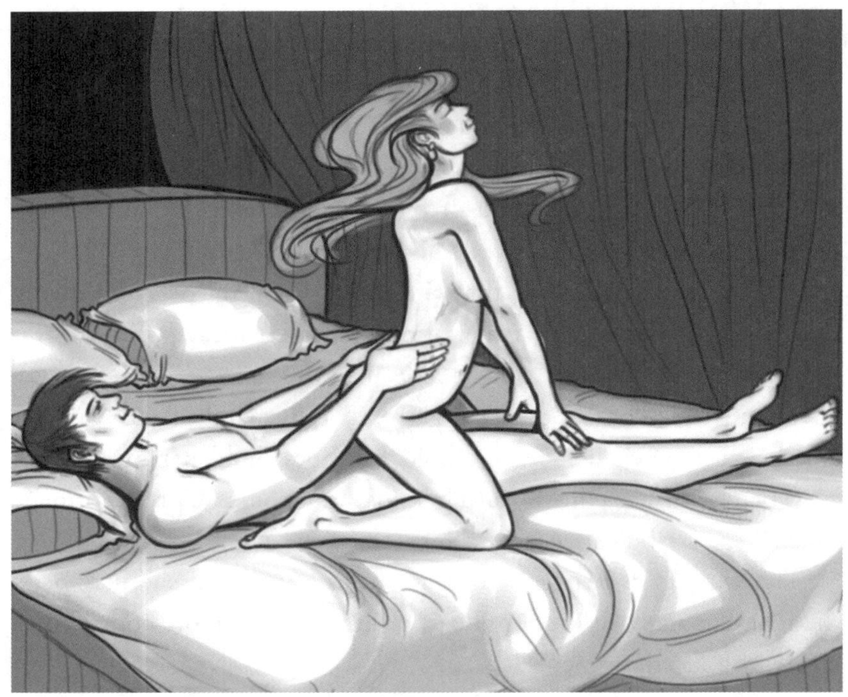

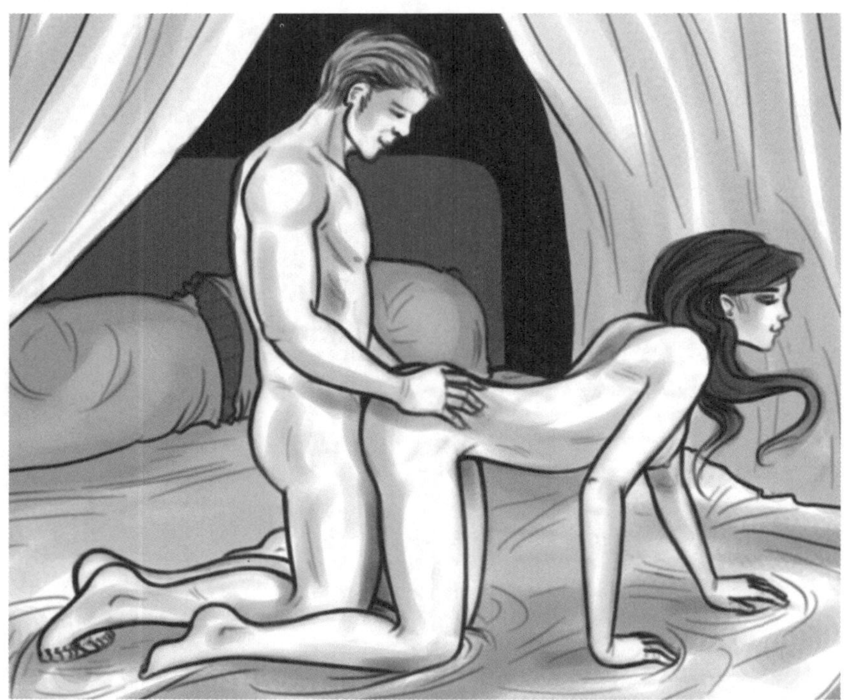

Another variation is when she turns the other way and sits on her husband while facing his knees. Doing so will give the husband the opportunity either to touch her back or play with her hair while they are having sexual intercourse.

The wife sitting on top of her husband on a chair is a highly arousing position for both the husband and wife due to the woman being able to control her orgasm and for the man to look into the face of his wife and enjoy the look of pleasure and fulfilment on her face.

9.3.3 Doggy-style position

The doggy-style position is when the husband penetrates his wife's vagina from behind while they both face in the same direction. Variations of the doggy-style position recommended for both pregnant and non-pregnant wives are when the woman bends over, as in the picture, or stands on her hands and knees.

As with any other sexual positions, even the doggy style comes with variations.

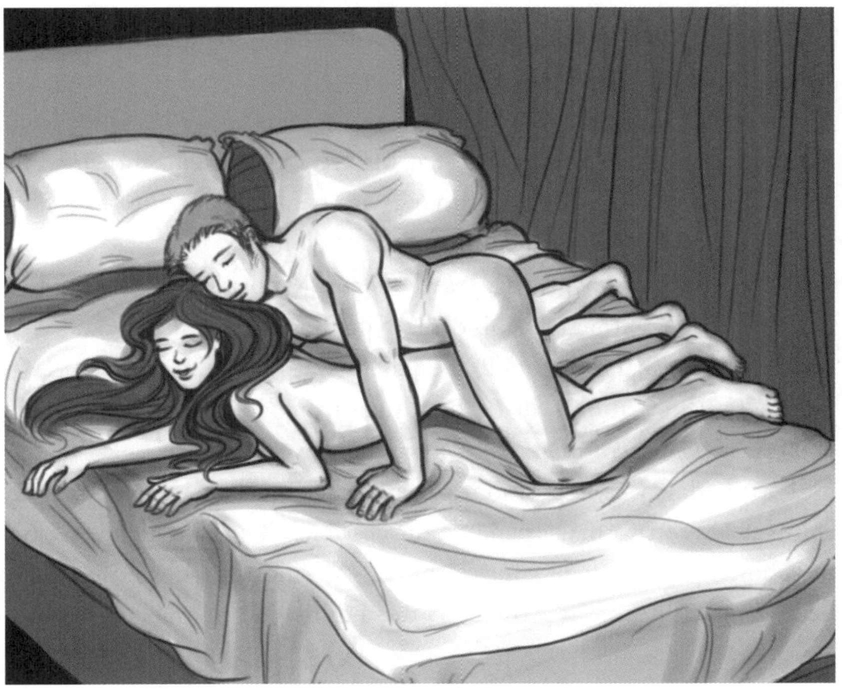

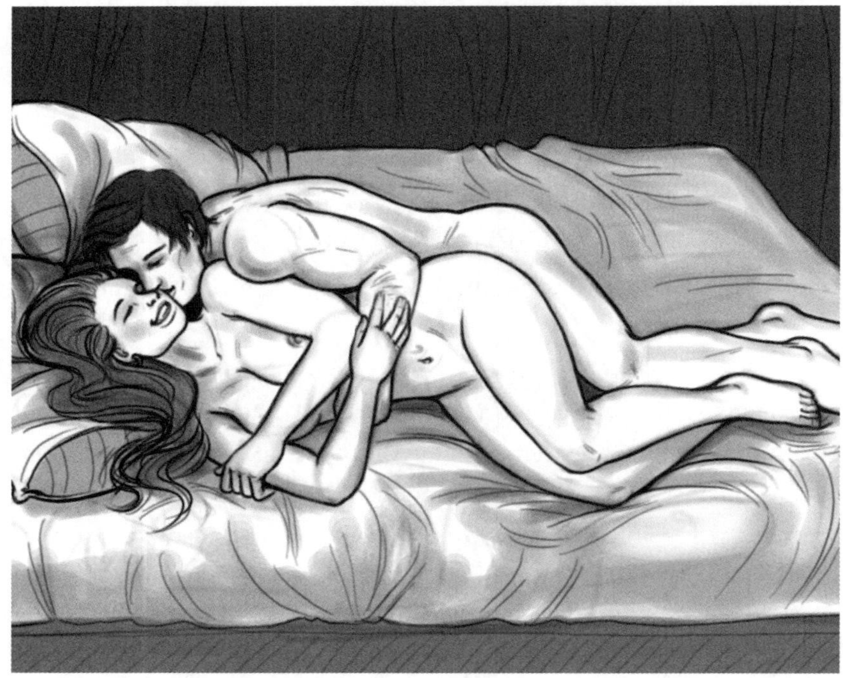

The husband and wife may lie down with the husband on top of the wife's back. His legs may be between hers or stretched over hers. Alternatively, the husband may sit up and even massage his wife's back and while getting sexually aroused, his erect penis may slip into his wife's vagina while he continues to massage her back and buttocks. This position is not recommended for pregnant women.

Another variation of doggy style is the K-position. The husband lies with his legs straight behind the wife. She presses her genital area against the husband and pulls herself forward, holding her knees to her chest. Penetration will be highly arousing in this position. This position is not recommended for pregnant women.

For the doggy-style position to work effectively, the penis should be completely erect to make penetration possible. When the penis is a bit too short or the woman overweight, this position might be more difficult, but with some practise even these difficulties may be overcome.

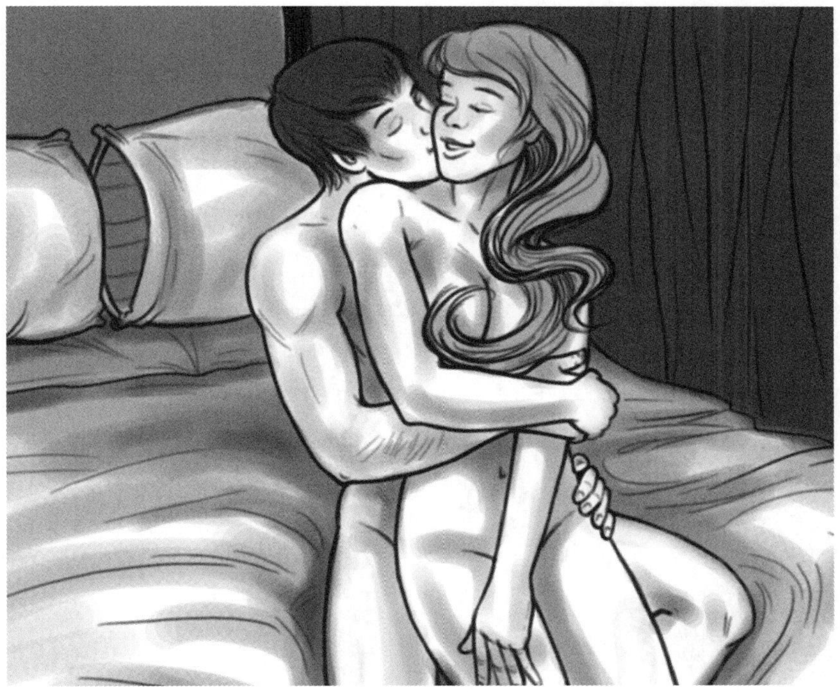

9.3.4 Sitting position

The sitting position is either done on a chair or even on a bed. This position allows the wife to control the depth and frequency of penetration. This is a great position when the husband and wife want to feel even more intimate with maximum bodily touch during intercourse.

Alternatively, the wife may turn her back to her husband and face the other way. Using circlular movements will enhance pleasure. Both positions are very intimate as the couple's hands are free to cuddle and maximum bodily contact is possible between the husband and wife. Also try this position in other areas of your home.

9.3.5 Standing position

This is an excellent position for both spouses to move freely. The husband can stand behind his wife or they can turn towards each other with the wife's legs slightly bent.

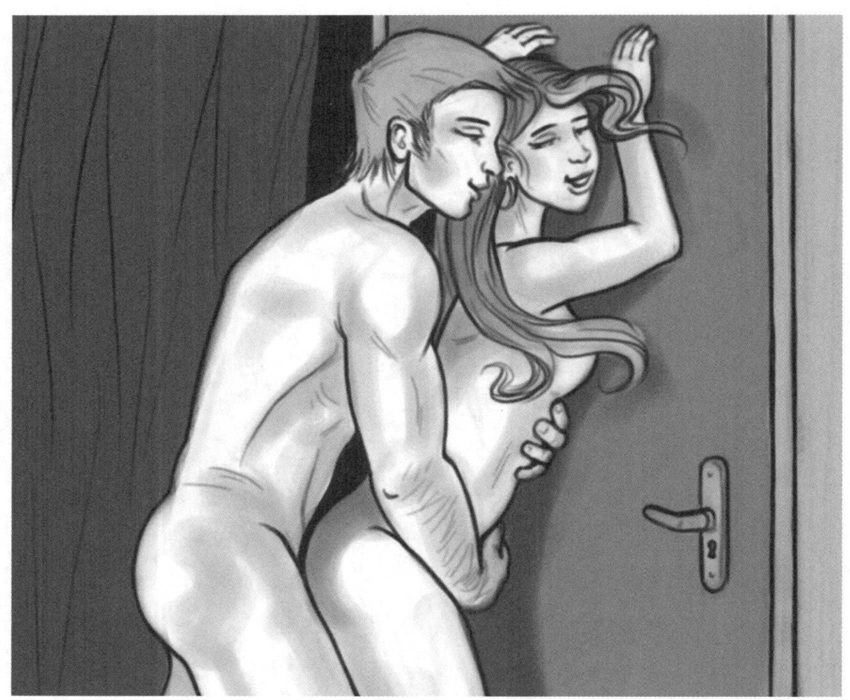

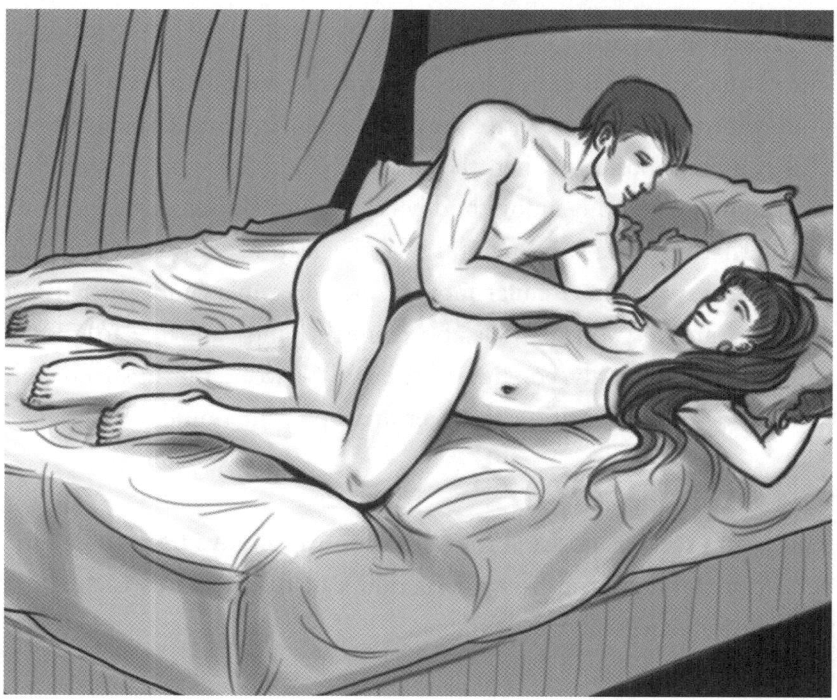

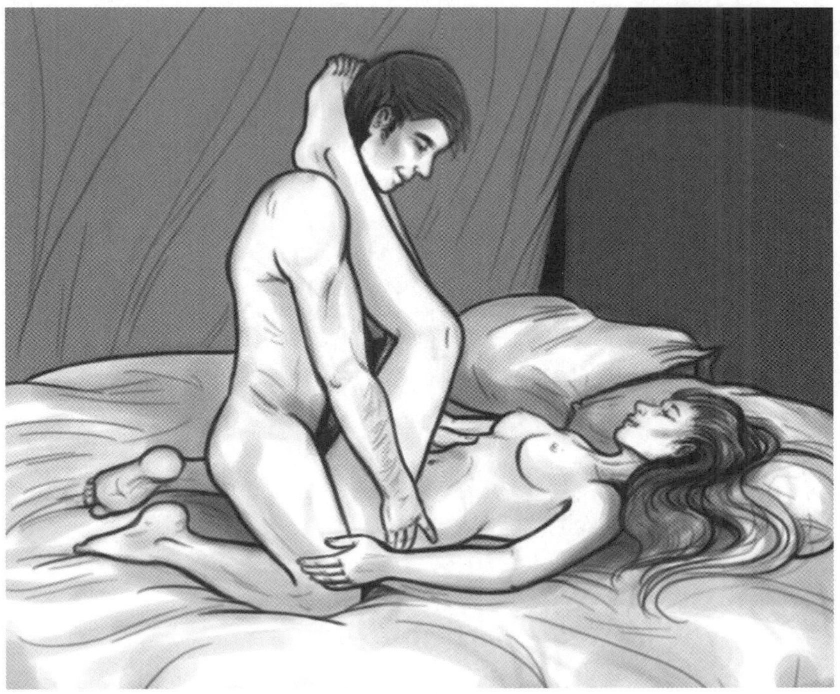

9.3.6 Man-on-top position

The husband turns his wife to her side and put his weight on his knees while entering his wife from behind. This position is very stimulating for the husband and relaxing for the wife.

A variation of the man-on-top is to turn the wife on her back, put her feet around his neck while the husband puts his weight on his hands next to her. This position is very intimate as both spouses can look each other in the eyes while enjoying sexual fulfilment.

9.4 Oral sex

The basic principle of oral sex is the use of one spouses' mouth on the others' genitals. Some people do not like oral sex because they do not like the smell or taste of the genitals, but when both spouses are clean and bathed, there should not be any bad odours and if there are, a medical practitioner should be consulted due to possible infection.

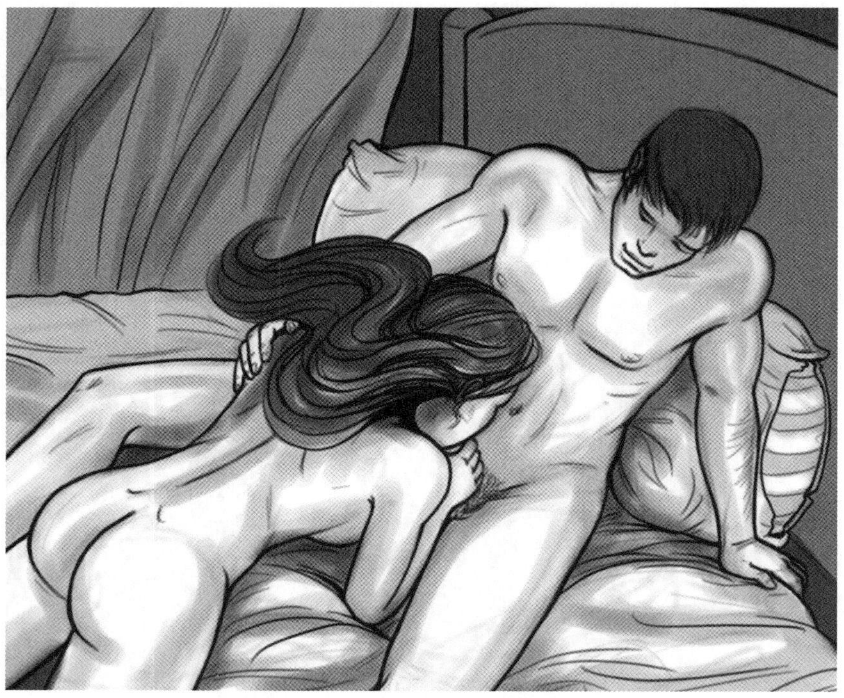

Oral sex is an excellent and arousing method of foreplay or it may be used as an alternative to normal sexual intercourse. The use of a condom during oral sex is a matter of choice or variation, especially when condoms with certain flavours are used.

Before oral sex, ensure all areas being used are without cuts or infections and thoroughly cleansed. It should be mentioned that a person with a cold sore on the lips may spread this herpes virus to the genital area of their spouse if engaging in oral sex and kissing the spouse's genitals, thus causing direct contact between the cold sore and the genitals. Rather avoid oral sex until the cold sore is completely healed.

Oral sex is highly enjoyable for a wife due to the direct contact of her husband's lips and tongue on the clitoris and surrounding areas. The result of oral sex on the wife is extreme moisture and enough natural lubrication.

Oral sex on the husband causes the penis to become erect for the purpose of penetration or to let the husband ejaculate for his own enjoyment, and this favour should be returned to his wife.

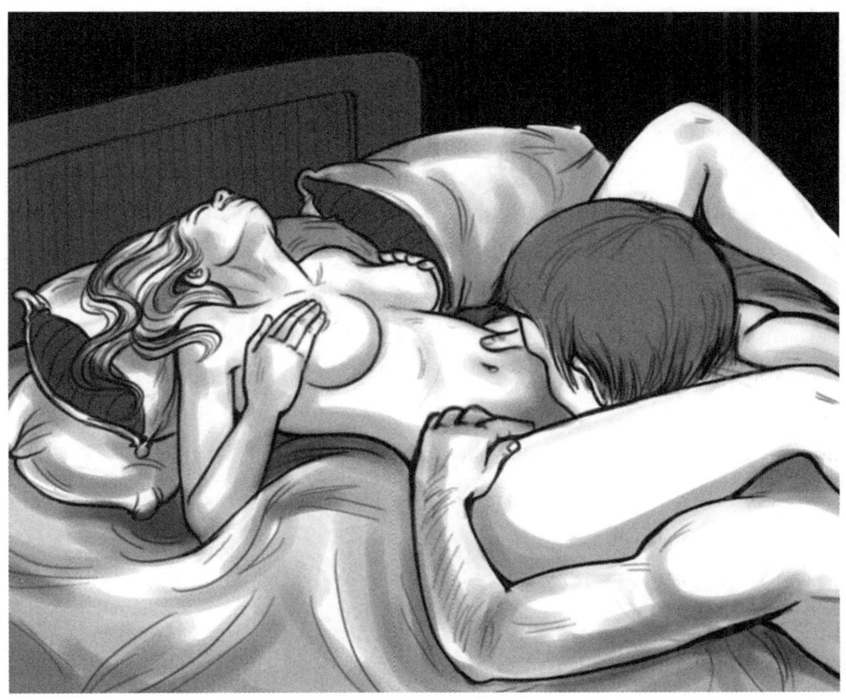

While he is undressed relaxed on the bed, you can move in between his legs and slip his penis into your mouth with one hand while moving your hand rhythmically up and down the shaft. The most sensitive part of the penis is the glans penis. To stimulate this part, move it rhythmically in and out of your mouth, sucking and occasionally licking in circles with your tongue. Use your other hand to hold the scrotum upwards, but do not squeeze. When your husband starts showing excitement, remove your mouth from the penis and gently caress his chest, stomach and pelvis area with one hand, then continue stimulating the glans penis with your mouth, varying things with your hand on the penis shaft, once he is relaxed again.

You can vary this process a few times, making sure he is uncontrollably excited and continue to let him ejaculate. The wife may allow her husband to ejaculate in her mouth, over her face or on her body, just remove her mouth before he ejaculates. This is really something you and your spouse should discuss in terms of making it a pleasurable experience or just allow nature to take its course and see what happens. Some couples stop before the husband climaxes and continue with sexual intercourse to climax.

It should once again be mentioned that oral sex is not about rules and regulations, but about enjoyment and what you do the first time may be different from what is done the next. Variation is always exciting.

Oral sex with your wife will be more enjoyable when you are both relaxed and the temperature in the room is acceptable. The husband can put his tongue on the clitoral area after kissing the surrounding areas, moving it in a round motion over the clitoris, occasionally sucking the clitoris and surrounding areas. Lick and occasionally suck at the labia majora and labia minora, going between the labia, clitoris and surrounding areas. You can use your tongue to penetrate the vagina, licking and occasionally sucking as there are several sensitive nerve endings located at the opening of the vagina. You may even lightly bite the clitoris, but be careful never to hurt or cause injury. Alternatively, the husband may lick from the vagina up towards the clitoris with varying speed, pressure and intensity.

Communication about this action is very important between wife and husband. While having oral sex the husband may stimulate the vagina by using first his one finger and then a second finger to spread the vaginal lubrication in and around the vagina. If the wife climaxes with her clitoral stimulation, this will contribute to a pleasurable vaginal penetration that may follow. Always communicate clearly about this.

When sexual play is extended, the clitoris can be stimulated again after about 10 or 15 minutes. This will in no way interfere with a normal climax of the sexual intercourse to follow, but may make it more pleasurable.

There are no rules; do what makes your spouse happy and makes it an enjoyable experience for both. It is just as stimulating to give as to receive oral sex.

Mutual oral sex is a very attractive and popular option, more commonly known as 69. This is done by both spouses orally stimulating each other's genitals at the same time. The husband or wife may be

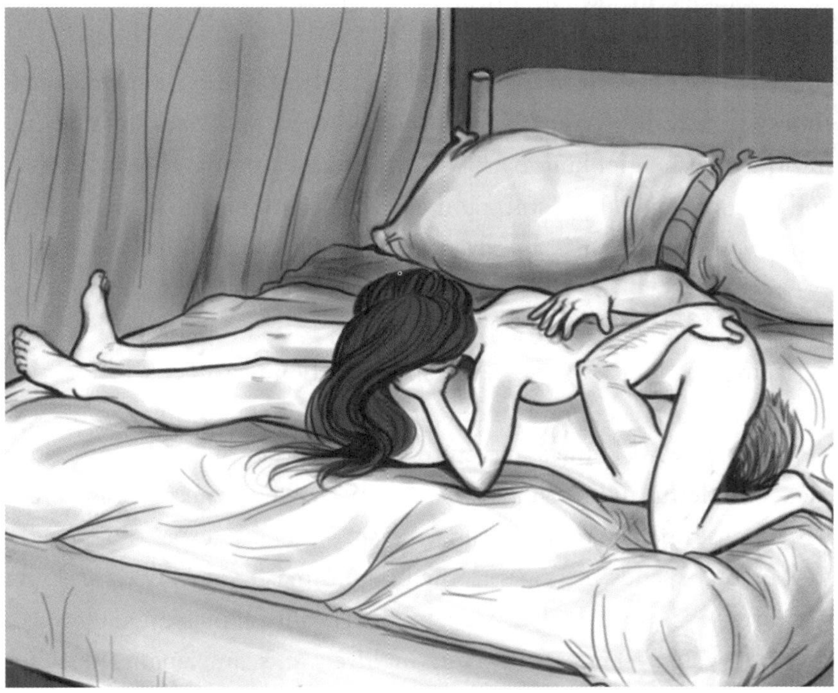

on their hands and knees over their spouse, lowering their genitals over the spouse's face for the spouse to be able to engage in oral sex. The spouse on top will then also reach down and engage in oral sex with the spouse lying down. Both spouses may not reach orgasm simultaneously, but try to ensure both of you do reach orgasm. You and your spouse will find the best way for you to enjoy this position when you practise it. This position is great because it leaves both spouses with hands free to caress and massage any way they want to. Try different ways and venues to please yourself and your spouse through mutual oral sex.

All sexual positions and actions take practise to perfect. Patience is very important. Even after being married for many years, you might find there is something you can do better or would like to try for the first time. So do not back down or lose hope or find that you are bored. Keep in mind both your and your spouse's ages as with age comes change in likes and dislikes. See it as an adventurous journey of discovery and rediscovery.

When you have been together for a number of years, you will sometimes laugh at how you began in the bedroom, so naive, shy and uninformed. When looking back, you will realise you have been learning and discovering and yet still stand amazed at finding you know so little about your spouse. It is an adventure to be embarked on daily.

9.5 Fantasies

Engaging in fantasies about your spouse is bound to get you to enjoy your next sexual encounter since it creates a longing for more. Some people think in words, others in pictures and so on; no-one is the same. The most wonderful thing happens in your body when you fantasise about your spouse and the previous time you spent quality sexual time together. The brain sends messages to the body to make you excited and give you energy, so much so that you develop a beautiful pre-sexual glow.

Have you ever seen a person in love? It is amazing. The wife's breasts become sensitive and aroused, her ovaries feel tight, her genital area becomes warm, the vagina becomes lubricated and it is like she breathes deeper and has more energy than usual. Some people start to whistle a joyful tune, some dance or simply have a great smile for no reason whatsoever, and some may even become clumsy!

It is absolutely wonderful how God created your body. The next time you fantasise about your spouse, think about how your body responds at the different stages of arousal. You may notice the palms of your hands become sensitive and some places even tense up, like your legs. No wonder some become clumsy! Your mouth may become sensitive and then your neck tenses. Think about how your body reacts to you becoming all excited about your spouse. At this moment, you may send a text message to your spouse to inform him or her about your thoughts at that very moment and you will surely receive a quick response from your spouse, making you catch your breath. It feels great to know your spouse is fantasising about you and wants you.

Part of fantasising would be to plan what you would like to do with your spouse. What you want to wear, or not. What you would like to do and how and when. Will it be in the early morning hours, afternoon, mid-afternoon, evening, late-night? The anticipation stimulates the mind. While fantasising, contact your spouse and let them know your fantasies, including them with you.

The perfect relationship carries both good and bad memories, and builds on the good ones to create an excellent past, present and future.

How would you have loved to spoil your spouse in the bedroom right from the start, knowing what you know now? Your fantasies may have become a reality earlier in your marriage, making your adventurous journey more exciting.

We are not suggesting that you engage in romantic movies or intimate worldly music, books or pornography for the purpose of becoming sexually mindful of your spouse. You are first and foremost a spiritual being, so it is important to keep your fantasies to those that God would approve of. There are so many ideas you and your spouse can explore, but keep your mind clear of other men and women; fantasising about your own spouse is an excellent way of creating marital and sexual excitement.

Has your wife picked up weight over the years or your husband grown a couch potato tummy? Ignore that and find in your spouse that which you like. Fantasise about her cute toes rubbing enticingly against your formal business pants, or his naked feet and handsome, sexy smile while he is cooking dinner in only his denim apron. God gave you an imagination with which to enjoy your marriage, so use your creativity to make your sexual life what you want it to become.

Become a hopeless romantic. Life is romantic if you see the beauty in it; God has created plenty of beautiful and perfect opportunities. You may spend your fantasy time saying to God something like: 'Lord, You know that tonight I am going to honour You by enjoying the love and the gift of the spouse You have given me. Thank You, Father, thank You, Jesus. Holy Spirit, please teach me and guide me. Amen.'

Ask God to build your fantasy life to include your spouse, and ask the Holy Spirit to teach and guide you.

9.6 Lubrication

What is lubrication? Lubrication is a fluid or gel-like substance produced by the genital area to reduce friction on the penis, vagina or other body parts. This lubrication can be naturally produced by the body or a fabricated substitute can be purchased, which will be able to assist in sexual intercourse if you are experiencing vaginal dryness. You can buy a lubrication substance at a pharmacy and some might be available at supermarkets. Be sure to buy a water-based lubricant.

Lubrication should not be confused with herbal oils or massage oils. Any oil-based lubricants are not as efficient. Lubrication fluids are usually water- or silicone-based. Please do not insert water or fluids into the vagina for the purpose of lubrication as this is dangerous.

9.6.1 Natural lubrication

Our bodies produce natural lubrication in the genital area to prepare us for sexual intercourse. This usually takes place during foreplay when a person gets sexually aroused.

Different bodies create different quantities of lubrication but it is all natural. So if your body creates lots of lubrication, you are normal and if your body creates little lubrication, you are normal. The lubrication glands are located on the sides of the vaginal opening.

Natural lubrication might be influenced by medication which might cause dryness; so does ageing, as well as traumatic events and fear.

Wet sex is good sex, so if your body does not produce enough lubrication, either find the cause and eliminate it or buy a synthetic product to assist in sexual intercourse.

9.6.2 Purchased lubrication

If you are experiencing difficulty producing enough natural lubrication, you should buy a product like a water or gel-based lubricant, making it possible for you not only to have sex, but also to enjoy sex. Sufficient lubrication makes sex enjoyable and assists in reaching an orgasm.

9.7 Summary

The Lord has given you so many ways to enjoy your sex life, and it is wonderful to think of how you can bring old ways back to great use and create new ways together.

Your sex life should never become boring and something to see as a household chore or as something to avoid. When sex is enjoyable and exciting, you will want to have more quantity and quality sex and, in the process, make your spouse the happiest person alive.

Never rush sex, but take enough time with foreplay to prepare both of you for sexual intercourse, making it possible for you both to reach orgasm. When only one spouse regularly has an orgasm, it is no wonder that the other spouse will begin to avoid sex. Not allowing your spouse the opportunity to also reach orgasm is selfish.

Make sex enjoyable for you both.

There are numerous sexual positions to try out and many variations of each position; it should keep you busy for quite some time! By exploring each other's bodies and making use of different sexual positions in different ways and at different venues, you will experience new excitement in your sexual lives. Do not get stuck in a groove; make sex exciting and adventurous. Try new things in the bedroom or outside the bedroom, but have great sexual encounters with your spouse.

There should not be any rules and regulations to follow when sex is taking place between spouses within the confines of their marriage. Just let go and enjoy it. Become a sexual explorer. When you have reached the place where you think you know everything, then it is most certainly time to start over again!

God created sex for spouses to enjoy within the safe boundaries of their marriage. It is so wonderful to think how free you are and that nothing can prevent you from being the wonderful sexual being you are. Make great memories to cherish for the rest of your lives.

Sex should not be a casual encounter between strangers. Sexually satisfying your spouse after many years of marriage is not only possible, but it is what is supposed to happen and that is what makes you a great husband or a great wife.

This is possible if both you and your spouse invest in your marriage to make it work no matter what. To do so, give yourself permission to be courageously spontaneous and become adventurous in the bedroom by trying new things and experimenting with new sexual positions; you might be surprised how sexually fulfilled you both become, and then you will know the reason behind the smile of your spouse when he or she leaves for work.

When you are sexually fulfilled in your marriage, you will never be tempted to look elsewhere for sexual pleasures and you will be able to stay true to your spouse. It is your responsibility to not get involved with a third party and have an extramarital affair and, since it is your responsibility, you should actively engage in romance with your spouse to ensure you are both sexually fulfilled.

If you are sexually unfulfilled, rectify the matter and do not give up until it has been dealt with. Take responsibility for being or becoming sexually fulfilled within your marriage.

CHAPTER 10

Sexual dysfunction

Sexual dysfunction refers to the inability to have orgasmic or sexually fulfilling sex due to physical or psychological reasons. Health-related conditions, psychosomatic conditions or surgery can also cause sexual dysfunction.

Whatever the reason for sexual dysfunction, it is always demoralising. It discourages sexual intercourse and puts an unnecessary damper on sex and sexuality. Sexual dysfunction is an obstacle to sexuality, but definitely a conquerable one.

Sexual dysfunction is often accompanied by embarrassment, shamefulness, a feeling of failure and sometimes even guilt. It is a concern not only for the spouse experiencing the dysfunction, but also for the spouse who is directly affected by it. As a result of this hindrance, sex turns into hard work and spouses begin to avoid it in order to eliminate the negative feelings accompanying unfulfilled sexual intercourse. Eventually it results in your inner passion being suppressed along with your spouse's.

But sexual dysfunction is not the end of the road for your sexual fulfilment; it is just a hurdle to be overcome. If you are the one experiencing sexual dysfunction, stop seeing yourself as a failure or thinking negatively about your sexuality. There is a breakthrough available for you and it all starts with the way you view yourself.

If you are the one being affected by your spouse's sexual dysfunction, it is your responsibility to not speak negatively towards your spouse about the matter. Lovingly, caringly and patiently support and assist your spouse to overcome this problem, and it will result in both you and your spouse reaping the benefits of having an unleashed inner passion again while experiencing sexual fulfilment. Triumphing over sexual dysfunction is possible, but it takes patience and support. Never make your spouse feel guilty about the sexual dysfunction and never break down your spouse's self-image and ability.

Try not to constantly focus on the sexual dysfunction because it will only lead to sex becoming a chore.

The healthier option is to keep sex fun and adventurous and not allow sexual dysfunction to turn it into something it was never meant to be. It is supposed to be a very enjoyable and pleasurable leisure time.

You may have been dealing with sexual dysfunction in your marriage for quite some time and you may not even think change is possible, but there is hope. Your sexual life can become satisfying and fulfilling again.

Be creative in your sex life; become adventurous and try new things while being sensitive and patient with your spouse. Stop focusing on the sexual dysfunction and purposefully focus your mind and sexual behaviour on relaxation and enjoying the moment, even if it is different in the beginning.

10.1 Premature ejaculation

Premature ejaculation is a sexual dysfunction where the man is so excited he is unable to control himself any longer and ejaculates when coming close to his wife. This is very frustrating for both spouses since the man is unable to control himself for long enough to make sexual intercourse possible or allow his wife to reach orgasm.

There are certain times when premature ejaculation is quite normal, for example, when a man has not had sex for an extended period of time and then when he comes close to his wife, he is unable to control himself and ejaculates even before penetration occurs or directly after penetration. This is not seen as a sexual dysfunction as it is a normal and understandable occurrence. In an instance like this the man should just relax and continue with foreplay and help his wife to reach orgasm as well, either by masturbation or oral sex. He may even be ready for sexual intercourse again after a time of foreplay.

Premature ejaculation is specifically referred to as a sexual dysfunction when it occurs every time or most times when trying to have sex. It is often more of a psychological reason than a physical longing for sex or his wife. Find out if you have certain beliefs about sex causing you to feel guilty or look back at what you were taught about sex and eliminate anything possibly being the cause of the problem.

Sometimes premature ejaculation is simply a matter of not being educated about sex and doing certain things wrong. The first line of action is to consciously control ejaculation with your mind. If the need to ejaculate becomes too strong, rather think about something to distract you, like your work situation or a house chore you still need to do or, if all else fails, your in-laws. Just joking, but you get the picture. Your mind has the ability to control sex and ejaculation so consciously making use of your powerful brain is the most obvious first step towards overcoming the problem.

There are also some physical things you can do to eliminate premature ejaculation. Some couples do not enter into proper foreplay in an attempt to postpone the husband ejaculating prematurely. The dilemma with this approach is a wife not experiencing full orgasmic sex because of not allowing enough time for foreplay.

Alternative steps to put into place are for the married couple to spend time together not intending to have sex, but solely for helping the husband to overcome premature ejaculation. This can be done through masturbation, mutual masturbation or oral sex, and when your husband is overly excited and ejaculation is coming close, then to stop and allow him to cool down a bit before continuing. Alternatively, just before ejaculation the penis can be squeezed on the shaft just below the glans penis or at the base of the shaft in order to prevent ejaculation occurring. When your husband has cooled down and ejaculation is not inevitable anymore, you can continue slowly. This can be done a few times and by doing this regularly your husband will learn to control his ejaculation and you will both benefit from the results.

During foreplay you can make your wife excited, but ask her not to touch you too soon. The glans penis is very sensitive and reducing touch on it may also help to control ejaculation as well as not to penetrate your wife too deeply when commencing intercourse. Leave the deep penetration for just before ejaculation later on. When during sexual intercourse the need to ejaculate becomes too strong, but your wife is not ready for orgasm yet, just lie still while your wife either still moves around or also lies still. If this is not helping, you may withdraw your penis from her vagina totally until you have yourself under control again and then continue. Effective communication during sex is necessary to solve this.

10.2 Impotence

Impotence is also a sexual dysfunction affecting the husband. It is the inability to get a hard enough erection and to have the erection last long enough to make sexual intercourse fulfilling and enjoyable for both.

Impotence can have many causes and if it is a regular occurrence, a good medical examination may shed some light on the matter. Impotence can either be caused by physical factors or psychological factors. Physical factors may include things like lack of sleep, lack of energy, stress, nicotine, alcohol, drugs or certain medication. Psychological factors may include wrong beliefs about sex, seeing sex as a sin, feeling guilty about not being able to satisfy your wife, feeling guilty for having an affair, stress, a low self-image, feeling burned out and defeated all the time or feeling like a failure.

Impotence is not good for the man's ego and it causes a vicious cycle to develop, where the husband is unable to get a proper erection and then feels emotionally bruised, guilty and ashamed, resulting in his inability to get an erection the next time due to his emotional state. His emotional state, for example, causes his impotence and his inability to get an erection on the other hand causes his emotional state.

This is very seldom a permanent state and impotence can be overcome, but it will take some teamwork from both the husband and wife. You should determine what is causing the impotence and then eliminate the cause.

If a good erection is achieved and it lasts during masturbation, it is almost a sure sign of the impotence not having a physical cause, but rather a psychological one. It should be obvious how fragile a man's emotions are when it comes to sex and his wife should not reject him when he approaches her for sex as it may eventually end up as the root cause of impotence if it is done on a regular basis.

When the husband is experiencing impotence for whatever reason, he will usually feel guilty for not being able to satisfy his wife sexually and become afraid that she might look elsewhere for sexual fulfilment. The wife should never make her husband feel guilty for impotence since it will only worsen the problem. She must not break him down with her words or make him feel totally incompetent and unable to satisfy her. She should support her husband and never compare him to other men or maybe previous lovers.

A man is very sensitive about impotence because he feels it affects his whole manhood. It is easy for a husband to become discouraged and feel like a failure as a result of impotence. To avoid this happening he should be made aware of his ability to still sexually fulfil his wife, regardless of impotence or not.

If a man struggles with impotence he can still sexually satisfy his wife by making use of masturbation, oral sex or even sex toys. There should be no reason for him not to still enjoy sex, but just in another form. By engaging in alternative forms of sex, the husband gains confidence in his ability as a lover and it will not be long before his erection returns in all its glory.

Overcoming impotence is a matter of love and support. In the beginning mutual masturbation may be a tentative solution for sexual fulfilment. A married couple struggling with impotence should become creative in their love making as it is a temporary issue. Your motto should be: Impotence is no excuse not to still experience an unleashed inner passion.

10.3 Loss of libido

Libido is the desire for sex and the desire to have sex. Loss of libido occurs in both husbands and wives, but it is something women experience more regularly. It is a lack of desire for sex and when you experience loss of libido, you can go weeks, months and even years without craving sex, seeing any purpose in having sex or desiring it.

As you can imagine, this is especially traumatic for your spouse. Loss of libido negatively affects a marriage because one spouse still has a desire for sex. If you are the one experiencing a loss of libido, you will have to compromise your own lack of desire to satisfy your spouse's needs. Even when you do, it may still negatively affect your marriage since your spouse will soon realise you are there without actually being there. It is not difficult to know when your spouse is not interested in sex, and when it happens over an extended period of time, you may take it personally and see yourself as the problem instead of seeing the problem as the problem.

There may be many reasons for loss of libido. Please note this is not just a lack of desire for sex with your spouse because you are having an affair and are getting sex somewhere else. Loss of libido is an overall lack of desire for sex.

Loss of libido may be caused either by physical or psychological factors. On the physical side it may be the result of a lack of energy or not getting the correct vitamins, nutrients and minerals. Pregnancy may also sometimes cause a loss of libido. Tiredness and busyness or being overworked and overstressed may result in loss of libido. On the psychological side, loss of libido may arise due to wrong beliefs about sex or negative feelings towards your spouse. Many times the main psychological factor causing loss of libido is fear of pain or being unsatisfied and unfulfilled by the experience.

Overcoming loss of libido may be as easy as getting some multi-vitamins and minerals into your daily diet or making an appointment for a medical examination. If you know the cause is psychological in nature, the answer may be as easy as making an appointment with a good Christian counsellor or therapist.

When loss of libido is evident in your marriage, never give up or become discouraged. The spouse not experiencing the loss of libido should never make their partner feel inferior or guilty. If the reason for the lack of desire is pain during sex, it should be handled appropriately; we deal with this in the next section.

If loss of libido in your life is due to not experiencing sexual fulfilment during sex, the solution begins with communicating the problem to your spouse in a loving, but honest and non-judgemental way. The next step is to do something about the problem by telling your spouse exactly what you need and want in order to be sexually fulfilled. This open communication then flows over into making the determined decision to have sex and showing your spouse exactly what you desire.

If you are the spouse with the good sex drive, take note of some of these inside tips you are getting directly from the one you want to please. Become creative and just let go while enjoying the experience. From then on make every sexual encounter with your spouse the most exhilarating encounter for both of you; then you are not only en route to overcoming the loss of libido in your spouse, but also unleashing an inner passion like never before in the process you are.

10.4 Painful sex

Sex should never be painful and if you are experiencing painful sex, something should be done about it to eliminate the pain. Pain during sex can be so severe it literally repels people from sex and causes people to consciously avoid it.

Some people find a little pain erotic, but that is self-inflicted pain and not what is referred to here. Painful sex is involuntary pain experienced when trying to have sexual intercourse. This is usually something the wife would experience rather than the husband, but sometimes the husband does experience pain during sex. When sex is painful, there is a physical reason for it and it is always a matter for concern. If pain during sex persists, a medical examination is advisable.

The most obvious cause for pain during sex is a lack of sufficient lubrication. Dry sex is painful sex. Lack of lubrication during sex may be due to not enough time for foreplay or it may be caused by handling your spouse too roughly or even violently. It may also be caused by psychological factors like fear, stress and even feelings of guilt due to certain negative beliefs about sex. Anger and resentment towards your husband may also result in dryness during sex as a subconscious way of rejecting him. A lack of lubrication may also be caused by medical conditions like vaginal infections, certain medications, birth control pills and hormone replacement therapy. When you pinpoint the problem, the solution will become easy.

Another reason for painful sex is the use of implanted devices used for birth control which may cause pain during sex. If this is causing extreme pain and making sex unbearable, seek medical advice, but the removal of the device and the use of an alternative birth control method is necessary.

Vaginismus is a condition defined as a spasm or cramp of the vagina.[57] This causes severe pain and usually occurs when the husband wants to insert the penis into the vagina. The spasm can be so severe it is totally impossible for the penis to penetrate and forcing the penis will only cause more pain and spasms. This is a psychological condition and is usually the result of fear or guilt feelings due to wrong beliefs about sex.

It is possible to overcome vaginismus if the husband treats his wife very tenderly and with lots of love and patience. He should make her realise sex is something to look forward to and not to be afraid of. A Christian counsellor or therapist may help with the psychological factors and the causes of the fear, and with the patient's husband helping his wife reach orgasm in other ways, they should help her overcome the problem together. The wife should enjoy sex and the husband should find ways to please and satisfy her to help put her at ease for penetration on a later occasion. Oral sex, masturbation and mutual masturbation may help in this instance.

If you are experiencing painful sex but are not sure why, seek professional advice.

10.5 Inability to experience orgasm

The inability to experience orgasm is something women may experience rather than men; men mostly find it easy to ejaculate and thus reach sexual fulfilment without any problem. When a woman finds it difficult or sometimes even impossible to reach an orgasm, it is due to something negatively affecting her experience of sex.

Women should experience orgasm as much as men do and when it does not happen, investigating the cause of the problem is the first step in overcoming it. There may be different reasons why wives are unable to experience orgasm, ranging from psychological factors to a lack of knowledge.

When the solution ship leaves the harbour of indecisiveness, you have one of two choices: you can spend numerous hours trying to find the reason why there is an inability to reach orgasm or you can just face it head on and do something about the lack of pleasure in your life and make orgasm happen. The choice is yours, but trying to find a psychological reason for eluding orgasm may just waste time you could spend practising to reach orgasm with your husband. The inability to experience an orgasm may have some psychological roots and be due to wrong beliefs about sex, but eventually not reaching an orgasm is based on a lack of knowledge about yourself, your body and about sex.

Orgasm is essentially a physical experience although it may have psychological factors affecting the intensity thereof. To be able to experience an orgasm every woman should know her own body and know exactly what turns her on sexually and what excites her. She then has to make those factors known to her husband. Discovering the sexually sensitive areas on a woman's body in order to know how to turn her on is a delightful journey the husband and wife should embark on together.

Reaching orgasm is possible for every woman and it is something every wife should look forward to when having sex. Getting sexually excited but then never being able to find orgasmic release is not healthy for a woman; it is also a huge disappointment for her and may even cause her to lose interest in having sex at all. To avoid this she should actively desire to reach orgasm during sex and her husband should patiently make it happen through skilful foreplay and sexual intercourse.

When having sex the wife should try to relax and focus her mind on experiencing her husband's soft touch, caresses, kisses and foreplay. She should focus her mind on drinking in the pleasure of her husband's presence and touch, and sexual excitement will be inevitable. The husband should observe what is pleasurable for his wife and then focus his attention on making it a reality.

Sometimes wives do not experience orgasm because they feel guilty for wanting it so much and then rather focus on their husband's needs and end up being disappointed again. To those women we need to clearly tell you: your spouse will experience sexual fulfilment, so do not deny yourself the same privilege. You have nothing to feel guilty about and your husband will enjoy sex much more and find it even more fulfilling when you are able to experience an orgasm. When a husband's focus is on pleasuring his wife, he will want you to have the most amazing time and enjoy sex just as much as he does, so let go and just enjoy the experience.

Unleash your inner passion; relax, enjoy the whole foreplay and sexual intercourse experience and you will be amazed how enjoyable sex can be for both you and your spouse.

10.6 Surgery

Surgery is not so much a sexual dysfunction but rather a contributing factor in causing people to avoid sex, either due to pain from the surgery or because of the healing period following surgery. There are two types of surgeries influencing a married couple's sex life: firstly there is general surgery and secondly there is specific surgery.

General surgery refers to surgery for matters not directly related to a person's sexuality, such as surgery to repair a hernia. Specific surgery refers to surgery directly related to a person's sexuality, such as a hysterectomy, sterilisation, a vasectomy or a prostate operation. General surgery usually only affects a married couple's sex life by introducing a time period during which no sex should be engaged in, in order to give the patient enough time to heal.

Specific surgery is often feared. When a women has a hysterectomy or is sterilised, she may fear that she will have no interest in sex any more, while a man who has a vasectomy or prostate operation may fear that he will be impotent and incapable of having sex at all. These are mostly myths and you should spend time with a good medical doctor who will perform the surgery and properly inform you of exactly what will be done during the operation and what the consequences will be.

Mostly people's sex lives improve after a specific surgery, for example, after a man has a vasectomy there is no fear of an unplanned pregnancy and then the true unleashing of the inner passion takes place. This frequently takes the married couple's sex life to a whole different and exciting new level. The same is true with sterilisation in women. The physical sex will still be the same after sterilisation and the man will still ejaculate, and although the ejaculated fluid basically still looks the same, it just does not contain any sperm.

A hysterectomy in a woman and a prostate operation in a man often raise concerns of sex never being the same again, but this is not true either. After such an operation sex may be different at first and it will take some getting used to, but eventually you will be able to once again have a healthy sex life. These specific surgeries are not the end of the road for your sex life, but may just be the beginning of a new phase in your sex life.

The best way of overcoming your concerns about surgery and your sex life afterwards is to spend quality time with a good medical doctor and when everything is properly explained, you will be more relaxed since you will know what to expect. Sex after surgery should be clearly discussed with the doctor so you will know as a couple when it is safe to engage in sexual intercourse again and whether you may engage in other forms of relieving sexual tension with your spouse before that time.

10.7 Pregnancy

Pregnancy is not a sexual dysfunction, but a blessing from the Lord. We mention it here as some couples are afraid to have sex during pregnancy due to the fear of injuring the unborn baby.

You may relax; sex during a normal pregnancy is not a problem at all, but you may want to try out sexual positions more comfortable for the pregnant wife, especially during the last few weeks of pregnancy. If there is a possibility of a miscarriage or other related problems during pregnancy, seek medical advice about whether sexual intercourse or any form of sex during the pregnancy is advisable or not.

10.8 Summary

Sexual dysfunction is an obstacle some married couples experience regularly as a huge shortcoming in their sexual lives. Most married couples will experience some form of sexual dysfunction some time during their sexual lives, either because the wife does not experience orgasm or loses interest in sex or because the man experiences impotence or soft erections at times of high stress at work.

When sexual dysfunction is experienced in your marriage, you should be patient with yourself and with your spouse and work through it. Never see the sexual dysfunction as incompetence and begin to view yourself or your spouse as useless when it comes to sex. Work through the emotions and openly communicate your fear and frustration with your spouse. Together you should support each other during these times and help each other in finding the solution.

Never use sexual dysfunction in your spouse as an excuse to start looking around to find sex with a third person, thus engaging in adultery and extramarital sex. When your spouse is experiencing sexual dysfunction, spend more time with your spouse wrapped in love and patience while making it your goal to assist your spouse in overcoming the sexual obstacle.

When sexual intercourse is not possible because of sexual dysfunction, become creative and find alternative ways to enjoy sex along with your spouse. You and your spouse may still experience sexual fulfilment by means of oral sex, masturbation, mutual masturbation and sex toys. Make a joint effort to find sexual fulfilment in each other in the midst of sexual dysfunction and you will soon experience it disappearing and changing into a healthy sex life again.

The presence of sexual dysfunction in your marriage changes matters slightly and where masturbation is mostly discouraged in a normal marriage, it is encouraged in a marriage characterised by sexual dysfunction. What should still remain is the intention to keep your mind pure and only focused on your spouse during a time of masturbation so as not to engage in adultery in your mind. To practically implement this, come to an arrangement with your spouse that you may, for example, masturbate while your spouse is kissing you, touching you or just holding you and being with you during it. As an alternative to masturbation, you and your spouse may try mutual masturbation or, in other words, combined stimulation.

What should become evident in your marriage during sexual dysfunction is the love you have for your spouse and the love your spouse has for you, regardless of what difficulty you are busy overcoming together. It is in times of sexual dysfunction that you have to make the choice to allow your marriage relationship to grow instead of allowing it to break down.

Sexual dysfunction is not the end of the road, but just a stepping stone towards sexual fulfilment and the unleashing of your inner sexual passion.

CHAPTER 11

Sexual quiz

Complete the sexual quiz below and get a better understanding of who you are and what you want in the bedroom. This is a great way for you to get to know yourself better and for your spouse to understand you better as well.

Please note there are no right or wrong answers, but all answers are based on your perception of yourself, so be as honest as possible to gain the maximum benefit.

11.1 Find out what makes you a great lover

Score the statements below on a scale from 1 to 10 where 1 is when you least agree with the statement and 10 is when you most agree with the statement. Place your scores in the table below and when you have completed all the questions, add up your scores for each column and write in the total for each column at the bottom of the table:

    a.   I love taking control of our love-making sessions.

    b.   Whatever we try suits me fine.

    c.   I love arranging every move.

    d.   Performance is my main thing in bed.

    e.   Making love is great when my spouse follows my commands.

    f.   Loyalty is my main thing in bed, it causes intimacy and I like it.

    g.   I plan some moves in bed, yes, I love thinking about them before the time.

    h.   I am entertaining in bed; I love the spotlight and being great.

i. I am loved for my influence and control in the bedroom.

j. My feelings are completely set into the love-making session.

k. I go to great lengths to make sure that everything works perfectly.

l. Let us try it and be really good at it.

m. I know it is going to be fantastic, just go with the flow.

n. Relaxing is something possible to me, which makes sex great.

o. I am very creative and arty in bed.

p. I am demonstrative in bed, and that makes me a great lover.

Column 1	Column 2	Column 3	Column 4
(a)	(b)	(c)	(d)
(e)	(f)	(g)	(h)
(i)	(j)	(k)	(l)
(m)	(n)	(o)	(p)

Interpretation of the scores:

The highest column total will be most applicable to you.

Column 1 = You are a very structured lover, knowing exactly what you want and how to get it. You can do just about anything as long as your spouse follows. You are the knight of the night, whether you are male or female. You can be excited with a sex life worth feeling great about.

Column 2 = You enjoy whatever you and your spouse do next; it is great. As much as you love making love, you love taking in every little detail possible. You are very sensitive to what happens to you while making love and you are very compassionate towards your spouse. You bloom when you are in a supportive position.

Column 3 = You are very creative in love making, you have a big heart and you are a very passionate lover. What makes you great is your commitment and dedication; the way you plan in your mind ahead every little successful detail. You are witty and fun to make love to. You enjoy making love and you know you are good at it.

Column 4 = You are great; you make sure making love works wonderfully. Your spouse loves making love to you and being one with you. You are most likely to be really good without putting any effort into it.

11.2 Find out what loving preferences you have in bed

Score the statements below on a scale from 1 to 10 where 1 is when you least agree with the statement and 10 is when you most agree with the statement. Place your scores in the table below and when you have completed all the questions, add up your scores for each column and write in the total for each column at the bottom of the table:

a. When my spouse touches me, I feel sensational.
b. When my spouse speaks to me, I feel sensational.
c. When my spouse focuses on me, I feel sensational.
d. When my spouse gives me something, I feel sensational.
e. When my spouse does something for me, I feel sensational.
f. I love being caressed, massaged and held.
g. I love receiving poems, praying together or whispering something sensational.
h. I love lying next to my spouse quietly for a while.
i. I love giving my spouse presents, even a flower or letter.
j. I love spoiling my spouse by getting everything ready, making a meal etc.
k. Holding hands and kissing is a fantastic way to make love.
l. Having a mature intelligent conversation turns me on.
m. Just being together the whole night, not even saying anything, is so great!
n. When my spouse gives him-or herself to me, I know they love me.
o. My spouse loves me when they do what I asked them to.

p. Touching my spouse sends shivers down my spine.

q. When I tell my spouse I love them, I mean it from my heart.

r. We do everything together and it triggers me sexually.

s. I like leaving presents all over our home for my spouse to find later!

t. I scratch my spouse's back, cut their nails, make them food, sit on top.

u. Hugging, dancing and holding hands while watching a movie is really nice.

v. I secretly wish my spouse would tell me how much they love me every day.

w. I want to make love in different places with my spouse.

x. My spouse knows I know what they like most, and I love giving it to them.

y. My spouse need not even ask, and I've done it for them already!

Column 1	Column 2	Column 3	Column 4	Column 5
(a)	(b)	(c)	(d)	(e)
(f)	(g)	(h)	(i)	(j)
(k)	(l)	(m)	(n)	(o)
(p)	(q)	(r)	(s)	(t)
(u)	(v)	(w)	(x)	(y)

Interpretation of the scores:

The highest column total will be most applicable to you. Take into consideration the fact that you have certain ways of loving which might be stronger than other ways, but all the ways of loving are available to us and applicable in some form to each person. The column with the highest score is your strongest way of loving and the one with the lowest score is your weakest way of loving.

Column 1 = You absolutely love it when your spouse cuddles with you and holds you, caressing them right back. You are a complete romantic and a very sensational lover!

Column 2 = Your ears and mouth are the two most sensitive parts of your sex life, you love hearing how you are loved, how good you are and you really mean every word you say when you tell your spouse how much you love them. You are a very sensitive lover with lots of love to give.

Column 3 = Your love happens when your spouse is around and proves their love to you through their deeds. You are such an intimate character. You love making things pleasurable for you both, doing all kinds of really special things together.

Column 4 = Let us wrap this up for you and give you the answer to how wonderful you are! You have a heart of gold and you are a very adventurous lover to your spouse. Keep it up and keep on creating all those adventures!

Column 5 = You have done it all! You are great in bed because you do those things worth doing. Loving humbly, the way you do, is a great gift, so keep it up!

11.3 Find out what your sense of loving is

Score the statements below on a scale from 1 to 10 where 1 is when you least agree with the statement and 10 is when you most agree with the statement. Place your scores in the table below and when you have completed all the questions, add up your scores for each column and write in the total for each column at the bottom of the table:

a. My spouse's deodorant is overpowering to me, I love it!
b. Whispering in my ear gives me a sexual rush down my spine!
c. Tasting and licking my spouse's skin is wonderful!
d. I sweep my hands over my spouse; they become electrified when I do this!

e. My eyes are the windows to every nerve ending in my system, just looking is sensational!

f. I walk through our home, smelling the food, the bed, the bath, my spouse's skin.

g. I listen to every breath my spouse takes while we engage in foreplay.

h. I love nibbling at my spouse's fingers, earlobes, toes and neck; it tastes wonderful.

i. Sometimes I just rub my hands over my spouse's body and passion fills me.

j. Looking at my spouse, every little tiny detail turns me on.

k. I have a heart-stopping moment when I find my spouse smelling me!

l. When my spouse hears what I am saying and listens, I feel incredibly special!

m. Sensation fills me when I feel my spouse's tongue against my body!

n. When my spouse's hands touch me I can feel myself becoming one with my spouse.

o. I have an intense sexual moment when we look each other in the eyes!

Column 1	Column 2	Column 3	Column 4	Column 5
(a)	(b)	(c)	(d)	(e)
(f)	(g)	(h)	(i)	(j)
(k)	(l)	(m)	(n)	(o)

Interpretation of the scores:

The column with the highest score is your strongest sense of loving and the one with the lowest score is your weakest sense of loving.

Column 1 = Your nose is the secret to your sense of loving.

Use it to love your spouse with and ask them to smell you in sensitive areas on your body as well. Go with your spouse when purchasing fragrances.

Column 2 = Your ears are the secret medium of loving on your body. Use them between you and your spouse to be blessed sexually. Also ask your spouse to say things to you that are nice, to whisper or to breathe aloud or use sound while being sexual. You love it when your spouse is loud during sexual intercourse.

Column 3 = Your tongue is your secret way of loving. You love exploring with your mouth and tongue everywhere on your spouse's body. Tell them how wonderful the Lord made them and continue to explore. You absolutely love French kissing.

Column 4 = Your hands and skin are intricately linked together to feel every curve and sensational movement of your spouse. Feel the way they move; feel and enjoy your touch and how they enjoy touching you. Touching is very important to you and therefore you feel loved when being touched and you show your love by touching your spouse.

Column 5 = Your eyes are your way of loving sexually. You love looking at what your spouse is doing and how they are doing it. Body language is very important to you. Keeping your eyes open while French kissing or during sexual intercourse, looking your spouse in the eyes, will send shivers up your spine.

11.4 Questions you may ask your spouse to build your sexual relationship and free your spontaneity

You can use these suggestions to your benefit. Try to be a great listener so that you keep learning about them. If something is uncomfortable to you, try not to laugh it off but mention to your spouse that it is a whole new concept to you.

- Can you remember how we fell in love for the first time?
- Is there anything specific that makes you love me?
- What about me do you like the most when we make love?

- Are there any positions you favour above others?
- What is your opinion about oral sex and manual sex?
- When do you like making love the most?
- Where do you like making love the most?
- Is there any specific thing that really turns you on that you have not told me about?
- Would you like to change anything in our sex life?
- What kinds of foreplay do you like the most?
- Do you sometimes fantasise about our love making?
- What about our love making do you fantasise about?
- If you had no limit, what would be your greatest sexual fantasy with me?
- Is there any way in particular you would like me to touch you when we make love?
- Are there any parts of your body which you would like me to touch less?
- When I am not sure about something in our relationship, can I trust you and talk to you?
- How do you feel when we talk about our sex life?
- When we make love, do you feel you have the freedom to do whatever you like?
- Would you like us to be different in any way?
- Have you forgiven me for all the times I made mistakes?
- Do you think we have sufficient foreplay before entering into sexual intercourse?
- Do you like a quick love-making session sometimes just for fun?
- Are you satisfied with the quantity of lubrication when we make love?
- Is there anything about your body you would like me to explore with you?
- Is there anything in particular you would like us to do every time we make love?
- Are there any specific sexual thoughts you have which you

would like us to explore?

- What is your idea of a perfect sexual relationship?
- What is your idea of perfect romance?
- What does intimacy mean to you?
- What does the word desire mean to you?
- Do you think we are having quality sex?
- Do you think we have enough sex?
- Am I discouraging you in any way to make love to me? If so, when and how?
- Do you have enough privacy within our marriage?
- Do you feel respected enough within our sexual relationship?
- Is there anything about our birth control plans you would like to change?
- Do you think my sexual actions are free and I am living out my sexual potential?
- What parts of your body are sensitive to sexual touch?
- What are the three things that both of us like the most about our sexual relationship?

Date:

Building great sexual memories

Your sexual journal

In order to create great memories, you need to write them down somewhere and what can be better than keeping a journal next to your bed?

What is a sexual journal?

A journal is like a diary, but you have the freedom of choosing when and what to write in your journal. You are not bound by time or days, but can just take it day by day. You can decide when you want to write down something special in your journal and what it is you would like to write about. The core reason for journaling is to track your behaviour, hopes and dreams for the future, and how you react to certain things; it helps to obtain an overview of certain facets of your life and circumstances.

You can use a few other places to keep some information available. On days you made great love, you may jot a star down next to the date on your desk pad at work. No one will know what the stars are about, except you. It can be fantastic, mysterious and exciting.

Write your sexual memories in a journal. Should you be a less private person, you might want to allow your spouse to read your journal. Take great care to keep it out of reach of the children and in-laws!

Bibliography

Anon. 2007. *Female Genital Mutilation* (4th revised ed). Online article: http://wiki.bmezine.com/index.php/Female_Genital_Mutilation, 2007-02-15.

Heitritter, L. & Vought, J. 1989. *Helping Victims of Sexual Abuse: A Sensitive, Biblical Guide for Counselors, Victims and Families.* Minneapolis, MN: Bethany House.

Herholdt, M., Knoetze, R. & Jonker, K. 2005. *On the way towards Emotional Wholeness: Self-counseling as enrichment growth and development.* Centurion: Dotsquare.

Holtzhausen, R. & Stander, H. 1996. *God makes sex great.* Vereeniging: CUM.

Holy Bible : New International Version. 3rd S.A. ed., 16th impression. Cape Town: Bible Society of South Africa, 2001.

Holy Bible : New King James Version. Cape Town : Struik Christian Bibles, 2010.

Holy Bible : New Living Translation. 2nd ed. Wheaton, IL : Tyndale House Publishers, 2004.

Kent, W. 1995. *The Greatest Love Storey Ever Told.* Parker, CO: TWM International.

Kent, W. & Kent 1995. *And God said Let there be Sex* (3rd printing). Parker, CO: TWM International.

LaHaye, T. & LaHaye, B. 1997. *Die Huweliksdaad* (4th ed). Vereeniging: CUM.

Scheepers, C.A. 2007. *Holistic Wellness: A Christian Omnibus for Whole-Person Wellbeing.* Lincoln, NE: iUniverse.

Tapscott, B. 1995. *Inner Healing through Healing of Memories* (15th printing). Kingwood, TX: Hunter.

The Amplified Bible. Grand Rapids, MI : Zondervan, 1987.

Wheat, E. & Wheat, G. 1995. *Intended for Pleasure: Sex Technique and Sexual Fulfilment in Christian Marriage* (2nd ed). Vereeniging: Christian Art.

Footnotes

Introduction

1. Wheat E & Wheat G. *Intended for pleasure: Sex technique and sexual fulfilment in Christian marriage*, p. 16
2. Kent W & Kent D. *And God said let there be sex*, p.1
3. Holtzhausen R & Stander H. *God makes sex great*, p. 16

Chapter 1

4. Ephesians 5:22
5. Ephesians 5:21
6. 1 Corinthians 6:19
7. Ephesians 1:7 and 1 John 1:9
8. 1 Corinthians 1:2
9. Romans 8:33
10. John 8:32
11. Romans 8:37
12. Romans 8:1
13. 2 Corinthians 5:18
14. Hosea 4:6
15. John 8:32

Chapter 2

16. Genesis 2:25
17. Exodus 20:14
18. Exodus 20:17

19. 1 Corinthians 6:17
20. 1 Corinthians 6:19-20
21. 2 Corinthians 6:14
22. Genesis 2:24
23. 1 Corinthians 6:16
24. 1 Corinthians 6:18
25. Ezekiel 18:20
26. Ezekiel 18:1-3
27. Ezekiel 18:20-21
28. John 8:11
29. John 10:10
30. 1 Corinthians 6:12
31. Philippians 1:20
32. James 4:17
33. Matthew 5:27-28
34. Leviticus 18:19
35. Leviticus 15:19-30
36. Leviticus 15:31
37. John 14:
38. 1 Corinthians 7:5
39. Exodus 20:13
40. Romans10:12
41. 2 Corinthians 6:14
42. 1 Corinthians 6:12
43. Ephesians 5:21

Chapter 3

44. Proverbs 4:23, New Living Translation
45. Romans 12:2
46. Philippians 4:13
47. Matthew 5:32

Chapter 5

48. Anon. 2007. *Female Genital Mutilation* (4th revised ed), par. 2
49. Hebrews 13:5
50. Genesis 2:24

Chapter 7

51. Matthew 5:32
52. Genesis 2:24

Chapter 8

53. 1 Thessalonians 5:23
54. Luke 10:27

Chapter 9

55. Proverbs 19:22 from the NKJV
56. Genesis 2:20

Chapter 10

57. Holtzhausen R and Stander H 1996. *God makes sex great*, p. 138

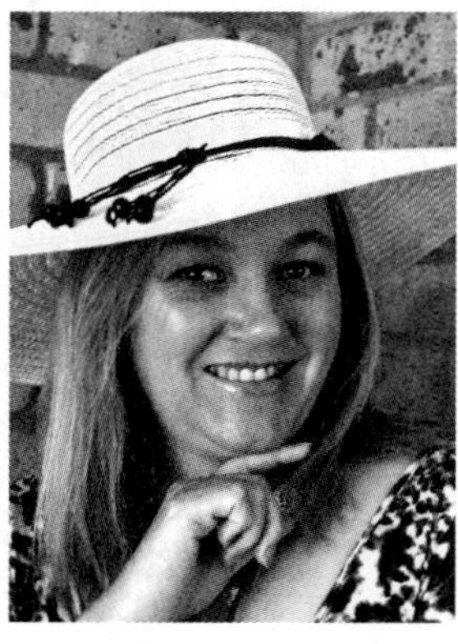

Dr. R. Dainty Shaw, D.Couns.

36B Rhebuck Crescent
Theresapark
Akasia
0155
South Africa

Tel: +2772 354 0429
Fax: +2786 614 3427
E-mail: info@drdainty.co.za
Website: www.drdainty.co.za
Facebook: Riehet Dainty Shaw
Skype: drdaintyshaw

Dr Riehet Dainty Shaw holds a B.A. (Cum Laude) in Counselling from Calvary University, a M.A. and a D.Couns. degree in Counselling from New World Mission Dunamis International University, and is presently studying ethnomedicine. She lives with her husband Joris and two beautiful daughters Vicky and Denise in Pretoria, South Africa.

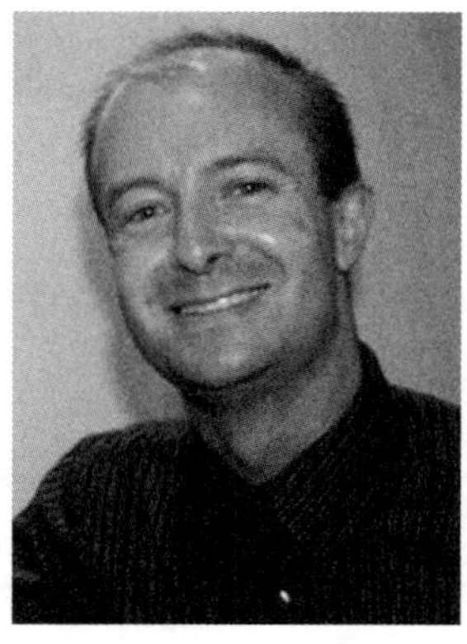

Dr. Christo A. Scheepers, Ph.D.

PO Box 3753
Durbanville
Cape Town
7551
South Africa

Tel: +2772 800 7243
Fax: +2786 545 8384
E-mail: info@christoscheepers.com
Website:www.christoscheepers.com
Facebook: Christo Abraham Scheepers
Skype: drchristoscheepers

Dr Christo A. Scheepers is a specialist pastoral therapist (trauma) and holds a B.Th. degree from the South African Theological Seminary (SATS) as well as a B.Min.(Cum Laude) degree in Christian Counselling from Theologos Institute of Ministry, a M.Min.(Cum Laude) degree from Commonwealth Training Institute and a Ph.D. in Interdisciplinary Studies from Commonwealth Open University, UK, and was registered as Doctor of Natural Medicine in the USA in 2007. He resides in Cape Town, South Africa, where he functions as clinic administrator for a medical institute and lives his passion of developing people and systems.

We would like to hear from you.
Please send your comments about this book to us at:
reviews@struikchristianmedia.co.za

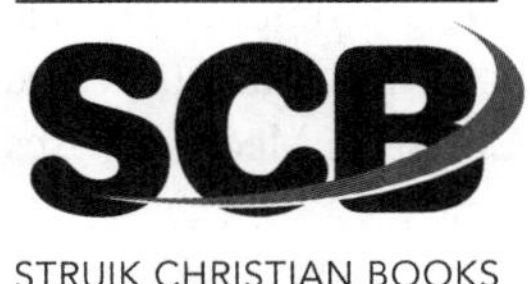

www.struikchristianmedia.co.za

We would like to hear from you.
Please send your comments about this book to us at:
reviews@struikchristianmedia.co.za

Christian Republic is a vibrant online resource website for Christians. It's a friendly platform for Christians of all ages, races, all walks of life and all denominations to interact and access cutting-edge resources online.
Main features on the website include:

- Christian Events
- Church Finder
- Daily Devotionals
- Prayer Requests
- Online Shop

Visit the online shop today at
www.christianrepublic.co.za and buy
this book and many other exciting
Struik Christian Media releases online.

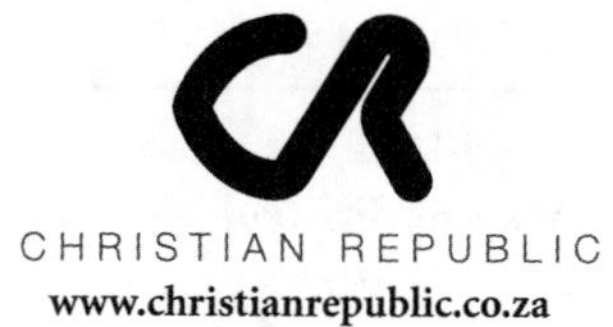

CHRISTIAN REPUBLIC
www.christianrepublic.co.za